WITHOUT A DOUBT

An Irish Couple's Journey through IVF,
Adoption and Surrogacy

FIONA WHYTE & SEÁN MALONE

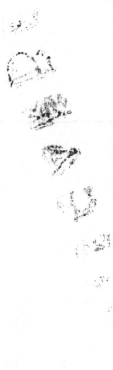

MERRION
PRESS

First published in 2017 by
Merrion Press
10 George's Street
Newbridge
Co. Kildare
Ireland
www.merrionpress.ie

© 2017, Fiona Whyte & Seán Malone

978-1-78537-118-9 (Paper)
978-1-78537-119-6 (Kindle)
978-1-78537-120-2 (Epub)
978-1-78537-121-9 (PDF)

British Library Cataloguing in Publication Data
An entry can be found on request

Library of Congress Cataloging in Publication Data
An entry can be found on request

Interior design by www.jminfotechindia.com

Typeset in ITC Stone Sans 10/14 pt
Cover design by Fiachra McCarthy

Printed in Ireland by SPRINT-print Ltd

CONTENTS

PREFACE

I have been trying to compose an introduction or preface to this book; words to explain our 'why'. I felt the book said it all, and then I came across this. Sometime after Donal and Ruby arrived, a mother sent us this poem. Despite the religious connotations, its message is profound and deeply meaningful to us.

A BABY ASKED GOD

A baby asked God, 'They tell me you are sending me to Earth tomorrow, but how am I going to live there being so small and helpless?'

God said, 'Your angel will be waiting for you and will take care of you.'

The child further inquired, 'But tell me, here in heaven I don't have to do anything but sing and smile to be happy.'

God said, 'Your angel will sing for you and will also smile for you. And you will feel your angel's love and be very happy.'

Again the child asked, 'And how am I going to be able to understand when people talk to me if I don't know the language?'

God said, 'Your angel will tell you the most beautiful and sweet words you will ever hear, and with much patience and care, your angel will teach you how to speak.'

'And what am I going to do when I want to talk to you?'

God said, 'Your angel will place your hands together and will teach you how to pray.'

'Who will protect me?'

God said, 'Your angel will defend you even if it means risking its life.'

'But I will always be sad because I will not see you anymore.'

God said, 'Your angel will always talk to you about Me and will teach you the way to come back to Me, even though I will always be next to you.'

At that moment there was much peace in Heaven, but voices from Earth could be heard and the child hurriedly asked, 'God, if I am to leave now, please tell me my angel's name.'

God said, 'You will simply call her "Mom".'

– Original Author Unknown

1

WHAT WILL OUR LEGACY BE?

On Friday, 1 February 2013, *The Irish Times* reported on closing submissions made during the final day of a landmark surrogacy case challenging the refusal of the state to allow the genetic mother of twins born to a surrogate to be listed as the mother on their birth certificates.

During the case, the judge presiding heard from a solicitor for the state that the Irish government planned to introduce legislation to cover surrogacy. It had been intended to publish legislation in 2012 but that didn't happen. The solicitor said the (then) Minister intended to take on board the findings of the Government's 2005 Commission on Assisted Human Reproduction, when introducing new legislation. As a consequence, Mr Justice Abbott reserved judgement in the case.

In late 2014, the Minister stated publicly that legislation would be introduced as a matter of urgency, and in February 2015 the Minister for Health was given the green light to draft the long-awaited and overdue legislation on surrogacy. However, there is still no sign of this promised legislation governing surrogacy or assisted human reproduction and worse still it has been announced that it is unlikely that legislation will be drafted within the lifetime of the current government.

SATURDAY, 9 NOVEMBER 2013, 11.05 AM

Aer Lingus flight EI381 descended, nosing through the dark grey clouds, and we looked out of the rain-streaked window, both excited and anxious. We craned our necks to see the first glimpse of land. There it was: an expanse of bright green fields all around us. It was raining heavily as we descended lower and lower approaching Shannon Airport. We were finally coming home, arriving into the best airport in the world; home with our family.

If we had known how our lives were going to pan out, would we have still taken the same path? It's a simple question, one that is asked by many from time to time. If we knew what the future held, would we seek to change it or accept the inevitable? Life is tough and painful at times, for some excruciatingly so; but it is a short life and it is our responsibility to ensure that we make it a happy life, not just for ourselves alone but for those who touch our lives however fleetingly. It should be a life that we exit in the knowledge that our children will be happier for our being there in the first place. What will our legacy be, I wonder?

2

GROWING UP

We were so fortunate to have grown up in Miltown Malbay, a small village on the west coast of Clare, where both Church Street and Main Street were our childhood playgrounds. The village was alive: shops, businesses and pubs thrived, all adding to the vibrancy of the village and creating the atmosphere of a bustling market town. There was no fear of abduction, murder or terrorism in those days. We left home at the crack of dawn each day during the long hot summers to act out our vividly imaginative fairy tales, returning only when we were exhausted and fit for our beds to dream up more adventures. We were both fascinated and terrified of the village's colourful inhabitants like Stevie Carty, Bid Behan and Katie Wak Wak to name but a few. Each one of them had their own eccentricities and idiosyncrasies, all contributing to our town's rainbow of colours. The population of our town growing up in the 1960s and 1970s was roughly between 700 and 900, and when the surrounding rural area was added, we had a thriving and productive population of about 1,600.

Ireland of that time nurtured a culture of socialisation and conversation, and where else would one have a meaningful conversation but in the pub. Even as teenagers frequenting the pub was a way of life, not necessarily to partake in drinking alcohol, although we chanced it on more than one occasion, but mainly to hang out with friends and play pool while we listened to our favourite chart hits on radio Luxemburg or the juke box. Seán and I lived just a street and four doors apart. We did the same as all the other kids, playing and gallivanting on the street or down at the sea swimming, happy and carefree. As teenagers I'm sure we were no different from others: hormonal, obstinate and giving our parents a serious run for their money. We were into the usual stuff, like looking forward to the next Fr O'Keeffe hop, sport and music. I liked the Bay City Rollers, ABBA, the Beatles, Fleetwood Mac and Neil Young, while Seán, well ... one could say his musical taste was a lot more cultured than mine, for he liked traditional, jazz, classical, rock and roll, rhythm and blues and bluegrass.

Sport played a major role in our lives. Cross-country running, basketball, table tennis, football, hurling and badminton all featured. Seán was quick and lithe on his feet, so he was great at running, especially cross-country. He also played both hurling and football, and to this day it's hard to put into words his passion for the game, particularly hurling. As older teenagers we didn't really mix in the same circle, mainly because Seán was a couple of years older than me and we went to different secondary schools. But like everyone else in a small village, we knew each other to see and salute on the street and have the odd brief chat. We did play in a mixed doubles badminton tournament once, but we lost. Who knows what would have happened if we had won!

With no less than twenty-six pubs in our village of 900 inhabitants, sure it had to be a way of life, one could even say it was our cultural duty, to frequent the pub daily to chat, to listen to music or at times, to murder a ballad raucously after a few pints of stout. There people would replay the previous weekend's football or hurling matches or just sup quietly, lost in time and thought for a brief spell, while waiting for the wife to return with the messages. Our growing up was in an era when a body could drive home after the pub without fear of being stopped by the Gardaí, and penalty points was in some way related to last week's match. The few cars that were on the roads were incapable of driving too fast. Traditional Irish music, song and dance were an integral part of our life. Fleadhs, festivals and sessions were the Oxygen and Electric Picnic of our time. Much has changed down through the years: the twenty-six pubs have been reduced to a more modest twelve; penalty points are now handed down at a great rate for those who care to buck the system and chance drinking and driving; emigration has tightened its grip once again and refuses to let go; and a fierce and long recession is battering us as we fight to keep our town alive, fight for its very existence.

Some major political events during the 1960s, 1970s and 1980s not only shaped our country and its future, but also who we were and who we became. 'The Troubles' – a common name given to the war in Northern Ireland – resumed in the late 1960s, and what followed was a period of serious unrest and conflict in Ireland. Some major events marked these years and shaped the course of Irish history: Bloody Sunday in 1972; the Birmingham and Guildford pub bombings of 1974; the Dublin and Monaghan bombings also in the same year; the Miami showband killings in 1975; as well as the hunger strike of 1981 during which ten men died. Events such as these were pushing the war in Northern Ireland beyond the realm of any realisation of peace.

3

ME

When I was nearing the end of my national school days, verging on that hormonal state while preparing for confirmation, a sudden and stark reminder of the fragility of our mortality was foisted upon me and my tight-knit community. While out walking one afternoon in early May with my best friend Mairéad and her brothers and sisters, we were struck down in an accident. When we least expect it, life can shuffle the deck of cards and deal the one we least want. That day Mairéad was dealt that card, and I lost my best friend.

When I finished secondary school at the local Convent of Mercy, I applied for every course under the sun which was what you did at the time. There was no points system; instead it was about who your mother or father knew who could get you into a job for life, preferably in the civil service. Failing that, teacher training or nursing would suffice. My parents must have known someone because I was successful in getting into nurse training, and in 1980 I went off to Jervis Street Hospital in Dublin to embark on my new career. There was no mollycoddling then. We went up on the train; I was dropped off at the hospital and was just left to get on with it.

At that time nurse training was undertaken over three years, and for us in Jervis Street Hospital, it was compulsory to live in the nursing home for the first year, after which you could move out to rented accommodation. After making friends we couldn't wait to move out into our own place. Sure we were young then and wanted to enjoy all life had to offer in the big smoke. It's the same today for any young student, but at that time certainly, nurses were renowned for their partying. We all blamed the unsocial hours and hard graft but whatever the reason, party we did. While both Seán and I had mutual friends in Dublin, our paths never crossed but once briefly. My time as a student was spent having great craic and getting into all sorts of trouble. One night, shortly after arriving in Dublin, I met Eamonn from Donegal. He had just passed out as a Garda and was based at Pearse Street Garda Station. While in Templemore he had become friends with a mutual friend from Miltown, so we all hung around together in the same circle.

Searching for a job in the 1980s was no easy task. We were in the middle of one of the blackest recessions ever to hit Ireland, with serious unemployment and major immigration. Pounding the streets handing out CVs was no easy task, but perseverance proved fruitful when I eventually landed a job with the Eastern Health Board. It was the start of a long nursing career. Eamonn and I were going steady and making plans to marry when another shock was to rock my young and carefree existence. My father died suddenly in 1984 as a young man of just 54 years of age. One word best describes my feelings at the time: devastated. I have often reflected since, wondering how my mother coped with losing a husband at such a young age and still having two young children at home to rear. Perhaps as a result of my loss, Eamonn and I grew closer and we went on to marry the following year. The years would bless us with two wonderful sons – Diarmáid born in 1991 and Rián in 1994 – and while I would have liked more children it wasn't to be. Throughout the subsequent years, I focused on rearing my family and carving out a successful career in nursing.

They say misfortune comes in threes. Maybe I just wasn't paying attention or maybe I was having too much fun, but life decided to bring me down a peg or two when Darina my beloved sister died at only twenty-five. Darina for those who remember her was full of life; she loved it and lived it wholeheartedly. But if she did, someone or something caused her to look at life through the bottom of a bottle. Someone or something unleashed her demons. Someone or something is responsible for her death.

My roots were deeply entrenched in West Clare, and Eamonn also came to love the area. Down through the years I always visited my family and kept in touch with friends from home. In the early days Eamonn tried to get a transfer to a station anywhere in Clare, such was our strong connection. When that didn't happen and when the children came along we had to put that idea on the back burner. Twenty-two years flew by until our differences became too enormous to overcome, and we separated in early 2006. In reality we had separated much earlier than that, but sometimes you look for ways to redeem a relationship or you deny that problems exist and ramble on aimlessly, directionless before confronting, accepting and finally letting go. Only those who have walked this walk, who have been through a failed relationship, can identify with and empathise with the efforts one makes to overcome the problems and keep the relationship from dissolving. In our case it was futile, and for me there was relief when the decision to separate was finally made. It was a very difficult time for us all but most especially for Diarmáid and Rián. If I have any regret, it is the hurt and pain caused to my two young sons during this period.

4

SEÁN

I was born in England. At least that was the tale within the Malone household. How we collectively arrived at that conclusion is anybody's guess because despite my very young age, we all knew, myself included, that I was born on 3 May 1960 at the Miltown Nursing Home on the Mullagh Road. At six or seven years of age, I asked my mother and father the usual awkward questions about where I came from and how I was made, to which my parents and siblings came to the convenient conclusion that I was born in England. And that was it. Or maybe it was the Ireland of that era, immersed in a kaleidoscope of colour and never exactly what it seemed. My father called me Peter, my brother Fintan wanted me to be called Michael and I was christened John Joe but ended up as 'Seán'. Did that fuck me up or confuse me? I don't think so.

We grew up in a very different Ireland to the one we know now, with its many societal changes quickly evolving in a drastically revolutionary fashion. We moved from horse-drawn farm machinery to the tractor, which I believe shaped an unprecedented transition of change. These lifestyle changes proved that time doesn't stand still. The worst manifestation of such developments was that people no longer had time for each other. This change would be evident much later in our lives, but for now and up to the mid and late 1970s our village was a magical place to be where nothing could worry or bother us.

The streets were populated with young families and the place hummed with commerce. Every second building was a shop or business of some sorts, all eking out a solid living. The country people traded with their town cousins. They delivered turf, spuds, veg, butter, eggs and griddle bread, the like I've never eaten better than Lizzie Brown's or Johnny the Doddle Connell's mother's special recipes.

There were a lot fewer cars then. In the late 1960s, at harvest time, I remember my sister Marion dragging me up the street to catch a spin on the back of Ja Sexton or John Flynn's hay float, all the way from P.P. Flynn's corner at the lower end of the village to the more salubrious part of town where we lived, before both farmers would ascend the hill of Ballard heading for home.

Fair days were regular and very popular events when cattle or horses would be bartered for and sold on the streets of the town. These fairs were of great commercial importance, as unlike the marts of today the sale realised on the day bore immediate benefit to the town. People spent a great percentage of the transaction there and then. Bills for the likes of meal and flour had to be paid for, men folk had to be fed and of course porter had to be drunk to seal the hard-fought deals.

Miltown Malbay was and is rich in traditional music with many well-known musicians coming from the general area. Musicians travelled to this area to study and listen to the music, as the style and approach was well recognised. This was well in advance of local piper Willie Clancy being celebrated through a very successful summer school established nearly fifty years ago. People still travel from all over the world to attend the school held annually in the first week of July. I was a late starter but developed my interest in Irish music by taking up the fiddle at the ripe old age of nineteen and later the mandolin and banjo.

I grew up in a house on Main Street which was truly open to everyone and everything. My parents ran the local cinema which doubled as a theatre for the many fit-ups and travelling theatre companies. The performers would stay at our house and they in turn introduced such colour, wonderment and excitement to our lives. My father promoted Maggie Barry, who cradled me in her arms as a baby I'm told, and Michael Gorman as they toured the area. He had Paul Golden, Bridie Gallagher and a galaxy of others, not to mention our association with circuses – Fossett's, Duffy's and Courtney's – all of whom are close friends of the family to this day. My father remembered McMaster passing through the town with Hilton Edwards and Micheál Mac Lomar in tow, and he didn't hold back in relaying colourful accounts of the shenanigans that ensued, but that's another story altogether.

My parents were republicans. Although my siblings and I didn't follow that path in immediate terms, developments in the six counties influenced our political thinking and direction in a very realistic way. From the sleepy village that was Miltown Malbay we were acutely aware of the conflict in Northern Ireland and followed developments there with great interest. I was deeply moved and affected by the hunger strikes of 1981 when ten men lost their lives striving for political status.

I followed a very active sporting career playing football and hurling into my forties. Sport was an interest I shared with my sister Marion. My father was very involved with the GAA and as a consequence so was I. I can say without fear of contradiction that I enjoyed every last minute of playing football and hurling, and to this day I really miss playing. We often left the cattle or a meadow of hay unattended in favour of fulfilling some important club fixture. The cattle never objected either. I suppose our enthusiasm must have rubbed off on them. My involvement these days, when I can find the time, is in helping the club in the background.

My parents both worked hard to give us the life we enjoy and what we have today. I always had a very close, open and healthy relationship with my parents; I was privileged in that respect. I can say honestly we were great buddies, and I shared every problem with them as well as the craic. My mother died in 1988 after a short illness to pancreatic cancer. She was only sixty-eight, and her passing left a terrible void in all our lives. She was a truly remarkable person and one of the hardest working people I have ever known. She had a tough life being orphaned at a very young age and out working in the world at only sixteen.

When Mam died I started a relationship with Susan. We planned to move in together and live in Dublin where Susan worked and where I also had work opportunities. So after working for a couple of months in Saudi Arabia, Susan returned home and we moved in together. The following December of 1990 we were married. We did a great deal of travelling before eventually moving back to Miltown in 1993. On 6 May 1995, our pride and joy, Tomás Padraig Malone, was born. We were over the moon with his arrival and settled into family life. Susan decided to re-sit her Leaving Certificate and then went on to university. Like any first-time parents we were blind to the delay in Tomás' development, but at some point in time it became apparent that something wasn't right. After a long journey with professionals and consultants, we were given a diagnosis of autism compounded by a learning disability. This news obviously came as a savage blow, but we strengthened our resolve to give Tomás every chance to reach his potential. To this day Susan and I struggle to that end, trying to keep sight of his needs, despite being divorced. Tomás has made fantastic progress in spite of the hand he has been dealt, and I am so proud of his achievements. My sister, Marion, along with Fiona, have been a tower of strength in their unfailing support for Tomás down through the years. Marion was also the sole carer for my father in his final years. He died in April 2008 after a great life packed with fun, colour and achievement. I am a happier person having shared my time with him, and as I said at his funeral mass, 'We did everything together but court women.'

It was back in 1979 that I started my employment with the Posts and Telegraphs or the P&T as it was more widely known, and ever since I have been involved in the telecommunications industry. When I took a severance package from the company, my great friend Noel Thynne and I formed our own small company subcontracting work from Eircom and today I continue to work at this.

5

TOGETHER

Despite what some believe, I would say one of the advantages of being from a small village is that everyone knows everyone else's business. I knew Seán had married, had a son and was now separated or possibly divorced. I also knew he owned and ran the Markethouse pub in town, which Eamonn and I frequented whenever we socialised at home. On those visits Seán would always stop by to have a chat with us. It's not that we were in any way special; it was just what he did with everyone. After my separation most of our close friends in Dublin didn't know which side of the fence to sit on. They obviously felt awkward, so one by one they all slowly drifted away. I was no longer part of a couple that got invited to dinner or to meet up with friends for drinks. Instead I was isolated and feeling abandoned. Friends I thought I had weren't there for me anymore, so I found myself visiting home more and more for both company and socialisation. Seán's pub remained on the hit list for a visit each time, and we started to get reacquainted. We seemed to click all those years later. It helped that we had something in common, both being separated and single again. It was good to talk to someone about all the shit that goes or comes with separation, just to stay sane during the dark times.

One night, when I was leaving the pub, he asked if I wanted to help him clear up, to collect the glasses he said, after the bar closed. Needless to say there was no clearing up done and the rest is history. We kept things quiet for a while. Maybe it was out of fear of what people might think, but definitely there was also fear that it might not work out, so secrecy was a safer option for the time being. I was certainly worried about what Diarmáid and Rián would think and of course my mother, the Irish mammy. What she might think was always at the back of my mind. I'm sure Seán was worried about his family too especially Tomás and introducing someone into his life. There is always the concern with a new relationship that it just might not work, and if it doesn't it is easier to make the break if no one knows about it. So we continued to have our secret trysts, enjoying each other's company while at the same time having great fun and craic doing so. We talked too much, laughed too much and loved too much if that's possible, and soon we realised we wanted to be together always. We had fallen deeply in love. Seán was slower to realise this but I knew he had. I think women are quicker off the mark in that regard. So for the next couple of years we had a sort of long-distance love affair while I continued to work in Dublin and travel to Miltown whenever I could.

In 2008, as I prepared to transfer to a new job, I was presented with the opportunity to relocate and work from home. Knowing the opportunity to relocate to Miltown Malbay would not arise again, I went for it. The sad part for me is that both Diarmáid and Rián chose to stay in Dublin to finish out school. It's not that they were rejecting me or didn't want to come to Clare; it was that as teenagers their friends were more important and they didn't want to leave them or Dublin in favour of the unknown. I knew at that age their friends were the be-all and end-all and I certainly wasn't in a position nor had I the inclination to argue this with them. I couldn't drag them to West Clare with me, much and all as I wanted to. So it was that on a cold November morning in 2008 I left Dublin with a very heavy heart to start a new life with Seán.

Because Rián and Diarmáid remained in Dublin I continued to visit frequently and they in turn came to Miltown to visit. That wasn't easy for them. It was always painful and difficult saying goodbye while longing for the next visit, secretly wishing they would eventually decide to stay with me in Clare. That wish did happen, but it wouldn't become a reality for a few years yet.

Seán and I built a very happy life and home together, but behind everything we were both hoping and longing for a baby. We talked about this often; we loved each other and the most natural outcome of that love was to have a baby together. Seán had always wanted a bigger family and for me, having a baby with the person I loved was the next step in our relationship; it would cement us. We tried desperately but nothing happened. I bought all the contraptions, gadgets and pills to ensure I was at my optimum to conceive, even trying out every food fad out there in the belief that it would all help in getting pregnant. Nothing worked. Ironically in the early days of our relationship and even after moving in together we were always careful to ensure I didn't get pregnant, and now we so desperately sought the opposite. Initially we didn't worry too much, but as month after month brought disappointment we realised we needed help.

6

IVF

We drove together to the fertility clinic on 29 May 2009 for our first consultation. I suppose for us it was an admission, a formal recognition that we were not getting anywhere the normal way, and we needed help. The clinic was one of those modern, bright and spacious buildings where the waiting room had the obligatory photo albums on display containing pictures of hundreds of smiling babies to raise potential parents' expectations. It worked; my spirits and hopes were raised immediately. I felt quietly confident that the clinic could help us. After all, we had both had children before so it couldn't be anything too serious, could it? In his consulting room, the tall, burly consultant went through our medical history candidly and then ushered me into the nearby examination area. He wanted to do an internal ultrasound. I recall lying on the flat of my back, legs in the air being probed by this man while Seán chatted nonchalantly on the phone, quite unconcerned. At that moment I could have quietly murdered him.

'Your eggs are too old,' he said, matter-of-factly. He may as well have been talking about what I had for breakfast. 'You will never have children the natural way.'

I slumped back in the chair, squeezing the life out of Seán's hand. I asked the silly, stupid questions that he must have heard and answered a million times before: 'But sure don't women older than me have children?', 'Isn't there a medication I can take?', 'There must be some sort of treatment that would sort things out.' All our dreams of having a baby were slipping away in those few moments. Seán, squeezing my hand tightly, knew I was devastated, and I knew he was hurting too. I missed most of what the doctor said after that. Why bother trying to follow the flow of conversation? It was all over. Some of his words seeped into my clouded brain: IVF, option, abroad. I needed to focus. I needed to hear what he had to say. Was there a chance? I pulled myself together. He was still talking about the option of IVF using oocytes (donor eggs). He explained that IVF was unavailable to us in Ireland because I was in my late 40s. Therefore, the best option was to go to a clinic abroad for treatment. The eggs could be fertilised with Seán's semen, and following an embryo transfer to me, I could get pregnant. An easy enough process, things no longer seemed so bleak. He recommended going to Spain and mentioned a number of clinics he could refer us to, including those in Barcelona and Valencia. Handing us the ultra-glossy brochure detailing all the proposed treatment and costs, he advised us to go away and read the information, discuss what we wanted to do and make a decision. If we decided to go that route we were to phone him back and he would get the ball rolling. In the meantime, he was going to do some blood tests so that if we decided to go the IVF route we wouldn't have to return to the clinic for these tests. They would rule out any communicable diseases, for example, HIV, Rubella, Hepatitis B and C.

Afterwards we headed in subdued silence towards the city centre, neither of us raising the topic. I read the booklet on the way and told Seán of our decision over soup and a sambo in a city centre pub. We would go to Spain; we would get donor eggs; we would use Seán's semen to fertilise; we would transfer the embryos to me and I would get pregnant – easy-peasy. It would cost us, but it would all be worth it. I think Seán got a bit of a shock that we made the decision so fast. In fact, he'd testify that it was a hands-up situation, gun-to-the-head job. But we wanted a baby together, and we didn't have time on our hands, so we couldn't dilly-dally. We either go for it or give up. It was as quick as that, and before we had time to rethink or change our minds I phoned the consultant to get the ball rolling. We only got his voicemail, so I phoned again the following day. I told him of our decision and that Barcelona was our city of preference. Accessibility was the deciding factor there because flights to Barcelona were operating out of Shannon. The referral was now made, and there was no turning back for us. That afternoon we became statistical failures of IVF.

Once the referral was accepted we both had to have a battery of tests done in advance of starting any treatment. These tests ranged from the usual blood tests to more complicated tests for genetic disorders such as cystic fibrosis. To us, while essential, they were frustratingly time consuming. We never dreamed anything abnormal would show up. My GP phoned on a Wednesday morning asking me to come in to her surgery that afternoon. I was working at home at the time and preparing to head to Dublin for a couple of days for various meetings. I told her I didn't have the time to go in and asked if there was a problem. She explained that a blood test carried out to check prolactin levels was showing abnormally high, in fact, four times higher than what it should be. She wanted me to go in to discuss this as soon as possible, so I agreed to an appointment on Friday evening after returning from Dublin. I admit I wasn't entirely sure what high prolactin levels meant so checked it out on the internet. I was shocked. The usual cause of high prolactin levels is a pituitary tumour. I trawled the internet to see if there could be any other cause, but it seemed not. How in the name of God was I going to be able to function normally until Friday? The only consolation I could glean from the information I had read was that a tumour such as this could be treated. But that would be all our plans for a family out the window now. The next few days passed in turmoil while I was in Dublin and Seán at home. All looked normal on the outside but inside I was shaking.

My doctor came out from behind her desk and sat beside me, and I thought, fuck this is not looking too good so far. She explained what I already knew. The high levels meant there was the possibility of a tumour. She had taken the liberty of booking an MRI for me for the following Wednesday morning and making a referral to a consultant endocrinologist. I cried that day. We knew the next couple of weeks would be very testing and difficult. We lived a surreal existence during that time, working away as normal or trying to at least, while inside we didn't know where we were or what we were at. Frequently we found ourselves hugging each other trying to offer comfort. Seán drove with me for the MRI scheduled for 8 a.m. It would be another week before results were with my GP and so the interminable wait continued. Exactly a week after the scan, the call came from my GP. She quickly told me that everything was clear; there was no tumour. Oh Jesus, the relief ...

But what about the high levels? What other cause could there be? Would this affect our attempts to have a baby? I went to the consultant who explained that while the levels were very high, no specific cause could be identified. Apparently although rare, it can happen. I would need to take medication to bring down the levels, particularly if I were to become pregnant, as the high levels could cause a miscarriage. Regular monitoring, MRI scans and managing symptoms, if they presented at any stage, were mandatory now. However, we viewed this as a small sacrifice to succeed in having a family.

7

BARCELONA

We first travelled to the Barcelona clinic in October 2009. Staying in one of the hotels that the brochure recommended, we benefitted from a 10 per cent discount offered to those attending the clinic for treatment. The hotel was lovely. Situated in a quiet place but central to everything, it was very clean and close to nice restaurants and bodegas. While attending the clinic, what struck us both was how clinical everything appeared. The building was spotlessly clean, modern and minimal in décor. Of course, the obligatory photo albums of newborns were innocuously scattered on gleaming tables and large-framed pictures of smiling babies adorned the walls.

After checking in at reception, we were immediately directed to a small office behind the reception area. It was the accounts department where we were asked to pay the due fees. This we would learn was the norm, and fees would always be required to be settled in advance of any treatment. The deposit of €1,400 was paid to register and then €5,000 to commence the process of sourcing an egg donor for us. It was the first of a series of payments we would make over the next couple of years that would eventually total about €30,000.

The consultant went through the treatment option open to us, just the one option. As he spoke, another glossy brochure was handed over with even more photos of smiling babies strategically located amongst the table of fees and details of the treatment plans. Our contract was signed that day, 27 October

2009, and I became patient number 10810898. We would need to quote this number in all correspondence. We were also allocated a coordinator called Nuria Pla. She would be our point of contact in the clinic, communicating with us and answering any questions we had. We had another series of blood tests done that day, and Seán gave a sample to be tested again for any abnormality.

Now the interesting bit: to enable them to match us with a suitable egg donor we were asked for our preferences on physical characteristics such as eye colour and hair colour. If we wanted blond hair and blue eyes then there was a long waiting time, however, if we chose dark hair and eyes then the likelihood was we would be much quicker in getting a donor as that combination is typically Spanish. We had no preferences save for a shorter waiting time.

Returning home optimistic and upbeat, we checked emails several times a day every day for any update from the clinic. Our blood tests returned all clear as was Seán's semen sample, now we just needed the donor. It took a few months before we received an email to advise us that an egg donor had been found for us and both her treatment and mine would commence once we had made the next stage payment. We received no personal information on our egg donor. When we questioned this, we were told that if we had a successful birth, emphasising that it would be after the birth, then we would then be told the blood type of our egg donor but no other information would be made available to us.

Life became a preoccupation of taking a concoction of medications at specific times of the day: nasal sprays, patches, tablets and injections. Simultaneously, the egg donor was also having treatment to prepare her for the harvesting. The clinic emailed the prescriptions for the medications, which were all generally available in pharmacies in Ireland except for the nasal spray. This was a high-tech medication that could only be prescribed by a consultant and then ordered in by the pharmacy. We chose to go to a pharmacy in Ennis for the medication. This was not in any way questioning the confidentiality of our own pharmacies, but was really because our village is so small and we were keeping everything close to our chests. We didn't want a single soul knowing what we were trying to do. Every few weeks, at specific times of the month, I travelled to the fertility clinic to have an ultrasound and blood tests done. The ultrasound was to check the lining of the womb to ensure it was thickening and progressing as it should, and the blood tests were to monitor hormone levels. This cycle of treatment and tests started two to three months in advance of the pre-embryo transfer and would continue after the transfer. If we were lucky and got pregnant then the treatment would continue for twelve to sixteen weeks, and if we were not successful then all treatment would stop.

8

THE TRANSFER

It went straight to my voicemail, so they phoned Seán one Saturday morning in mid-May 2010. Unusually, Seán was working on a weekend day and just happened to be swinging from the top of a pole when the clinic told him that we needed to be in Barcelona on Monday morning. Everything was good to go. The eggs were ready to be harvested, and the transfer would take place a few days later. On autopilot, I immediately started looking for flights, conscious that the short time frame would surely mean expensive fares. Sure enough, they were almost €1,000. Flights to Barcelona from Dublin facilitated our need to get in very early on Monday morning, go directly to the clinic and return home for work the following day. Despite concerns due to the infamous ash cloud over Europe, all went to plan and we were at the clinic by 10.30 a.m. on Monday morning. Seán gave the sample. The eggs would be harvested that same day, and they would contact us that evening with the details of how many they had retrieved and how many were successfully fertilised. Fingers crossed we would be lucky. We were both back at work the following morning as if we had never been anywhere.

They had retrieved eighteen eggs and following fertilisation they had eight pre-embryos. Two of the pre-embryos would be ready for transfer on Thursday as planned. We flew back out on Thursday morning for the transfer. We had taken Friday off work so that we could stay a few days in Barcelona. The clinic had advised us not to travel in the immediate aftermath of the transfer to allow the pre-embryos to develop. They seemed especially concerned about us driving in Ireland. Every time we met our doctor, he described his holiday in Ireland and in particular he talked about our winding roads, making circular motions with his hands, rolling his eyes and saying, 'not good, not good'. The ash cloud was still a problem, so again with fingers and toes crossed we hoped to get there in time for the transfer without any flight delays or cancellations. On reflection we realise we were very lucky travelling over and back without a hitch given all the air-travel disruption that was going on around us.

Thursday morning was lovely and warm in Barcelona. We arrived at the clinic, as instructed, one hour in advance of the transfer and with a full bladder. I had my water bottle to hand and a heart full of apprehension and excitement. The main reason we were asked to be there an hour in advance was to pay our dues. Formalities over and back in the waiting room, we waited and waited. Two hours passed and I just couldn't hold it anymore. Bursting, I ran to the toilet. Panicked I would be called with an empty bladder, I started gulping water all over again.

As we sat watching what was going on around us we saw many couples, like ourselves, in the same boat. It was easy to pick them out; they were the vulnerable-looking ones, sitting holding hands, stealing excited glances at each other, putting their dreams and blind faith completely in the hands of others. There were some men and women attending the clinic on their own. I presumed they were either egg donors, sperm donors or maybe single parents-to-be. After an eternity we were led to an elevator and up to the second floor where we were shown into a bedroom. Complete with en-suite facilities, high-tech bed, wardrobes and phone, it had everything a state-of-the-art hospital or clinic room should have. We were told to put on the gowns and flip-flops provided and again ... we were to wait. My bladder again was fit to burst and I found myself making another undignified dash for the toilet, only to start the gulping process all over again. Every time footsteps passed outside our door we kept thinking they were coming to us.

Eventually a nurse stood in the doorway and introduced herself as Nuria Pla, my link nurse with whom I had been emailing all this time. It was good to be able to put a face to the name. She led us to the theatre on the same floor, directed us to stand in a specific area and handed us disposable shoe covers to put over our flip-flops and disposable hats for our hair. We proceeded through two adjoining doors, one leading into the theatre where the procedure would be carried out and another into the laboratory where our precious embryos awaited. Another nurse emerged from the adjacent lab door and led us into the theatre. The room was tiny with an examination couch, monitors and trolleys filled with various pieces of clinical equipment. Being extremely careful not to touch off anything, I sat at the end of the examination couch and waited again.

Seán was sitting on a stool beside me when the doctor entered the room, gowned and masked. He explained that the laboratory embryologist would be coming in to check my identity and to explain about the pre-embryos and the process itself. We would be allowed to ask two questions of the embryologist and no more. If we had more queries we would have to direct them to the doctor or the staff after the transfer. The limit on the questions we think was more to do with time and the sensitive and delicate nature of the embryologist's work as opposed to anything else. He checked my name and details again to be sure he had the correct person matched with the pre-embryos, and then he quickly explained how they would transfer two pre-embryos. Both were excellent quality. We asked our two questions which he answered and then quickly retreated to his lab. Placing my legs in the stirrups at each side of the examination couch, I lay back and waited. Everything was projected onto the wall of the tiny room, so with Seán by my side holding my hand, we watched in awe as our embryos were placed carefully inside me.

Ten minutes is all it took, and I was on a trolley being wheeled back to the bedroom by the nurse and Seán. I was advised to stay in bed and relax for one hour. I barely moved so

terrified was I that I would do damage to the embryos. Again
bursting to pee, I forced myself to hold on for as long as possible.
The doctor arrived to give us photographs of our two embryos
now growing inside me. He also handed over a list of instructions
to follow as well as a prescription for painkillers if needed. There
was to be no excessive heat so that was the sunbathing in
Barcelona out the window! Other instructions included,
absolutely no swimming, no saunas, drinking plenty of water
and no alcohol. I was to continue taking the medications until
otherwise instructed, and if I started bleeding or felt unwell at
any stage, I was to contact him immediately. He gave us a date
two weeks from then to go to the fertility clinic to have the
BhCG blood test done. This would confirm if we were having a
baby or not. After the hour I could go to the bathroom, get
dressed and leave, just like that, so surreal after everything that
had happened. Well after the hour I was still afraid to move, so
we waited a bit longer. Even when I did get up I moved slowly
and deliberately, as if I had major surgery done. In the taxi on
the way back to the hotel I worried about every bump we drove
over. Wrecked from the stress of it all we slept for the next few
hours. For the remainder of our few days in Barcelona we were
typical tourists, sightseeing and enjoying Spanish tapas and
water! Seán sampled the beer but was forbidden to enjoy wine
with his meal. It would have been akin to treason and very
unwise of him to do so in front of me while I was limited to
water.

Our return flight to Dublin landed around 1 a.m. Both of us
were tired and faced a long drive ahead of us. We drove home
via Galway thinking it would be a better road, but it was worse,
as we tried to avoid all the potholes between Gort and Ennis,
which had been caused by the bad winter weather. Almost at
home, Seán, exhausted behind the wheel, started to nod off.
Jesus my heart was in my mouth by the time we hit Miltown at
nearly 5 a.m. We were shattered but happy and so very very
hopeful.

9

PREGNANT

Twelve days later, with a belly full of dreams, I travelled to my appointment at the fertility clinic. While drawing blood the nurse asked me if I had done a pregnancy test myself that morning. I hadn't. It hadn't even crossed my bloody mind. How stupid of me! The result would come back later that afternoon, and she said she would phone me. As I waited for the call, I fidgeted and paced. I couldn't concentrate on anything, and I became more and more anxious. I heard the ring and drew a deep breath.

'Are you on your own?' she asked.

Shit … it was bad news. I knew it.

'Congratulations!' she said.

I swear my heart did stop for a split second. I was pregnant. First try and I was pregnant. Whoohoo!

I wanted it to be special when I told Seán the news. I scurried off to a chemist, bought a home pregnancy testing kit and there it was – a blue positive plus. It's not that I ever doubted the result, but it just made it real. It made it more tangible to be able to hold the result in my hand, to keep forever and especially for the day when I could show it to our son or daughter.

But first, I wanted to create Seán's moment. I remember the day so well. It was a bright sunny day as we walked on the sand at the white strand and I handed him the pregnancy test. He just stood still in stock, looking at it and then at me. He was going to be a dad again; he was almost disbelieving. We hugged. Over the moon doesn't describe our happiness at that moment; life couldn't get any better.

Later I emailed the clinic in Barcelona with the results. Their response was congratulatory and professional as expected. Two weeks later we had a scan to check how things were progressing and to see if it was a single or twin pregnancy. We both looked at the one tiny single speck on the screen. That was ... our baby.

I went off alcohol and coffee. I ate as healthily as possible and got plenty of rest. I even stopped jogging just in case. We told no one. The Willie Clancy Festival was upon us when I was eleven weeks pregnant. Normally I worked in the bar for this week, as it was the busiest week of the whole year. This year, however, I didn't work at all. I did everything by the book.

On hindsight there were signs that something was wrong, but I didn't pick up on them. We were having dinner in the Chinese restaurant on the last Saturday night of the festival before going our separate ways. Seán was going to work in the bar, and I was heading home. We were talking about the fact that we were almost at the time when it would be safe enough to start telling people. We had a really good feeling about the pregnancy, so much so that on Sunday, bursting to tell someone, I let it out to my friend Emer. I know she thought we were mad, but she was also genuinely delighted for us. She was sworn to secrecy.

That awful day our world was shattered. I was bleeding. I phoned Seán in a panic, knowing that I was probably losing our baby. He raced home as I phoned my GP who in turn phoned the hospital and arranged for me to be seen immediately. Driving to the hospital was the longest journey yet, if that makes sense – I didn't want it to end. I was sick to my stomach. I knew we had lost our baby, but still I clung to hope. It was preposterous to be sitting in a waiting room – a room full of happy, pregnant women – watching as one after the other emerged smiling following their scans. Would I be smiling? Or would our worst fear be confirmed? My name was called aloud and only then did I wish I could sit longer in that preposterous waiting room. For as long as I was waiting I was still pregnant.

The nurse was very kind, and once she realised why we were there she apologised profusely. She knew it wasn't right. It was completely insensitive having to wait in a room full of pregnant women. It wasn't her fault. The facilities were wholly inadequate. She wasn't responsible for them, but she was the one apologising to us. I watched Seán's face as she did the scan, scrutinising his expression for that glimmer of hope. There was none. She apologised again. 'I'm sorry,' she said, and in that instant, our baby was gone.

The doctor prescribed antibiotics, painkillers and rest. There was a possibility I would have to return to the hospital in a week or so, but that would depend on whether or not I passed the foetus by natural means. Is there a natural means of passing your baby? I think not. Inconsolable is the word I would use to describe the following days and weeks. I wondered what I did wrong, what we did wrong and what we did to deserve this. The pain was immeasurable. All the questions, all the tears and no answers.

I contacted the clinic in Spain. They were also 'very sorry'. Instructions were uttered professionally; it was standard procedure. I was to stop taking the medication and they would arrange for a phone call with Dr Guerin to discuss 'what now'. I wanted to know the 'what now' immediately, not next month or next week but today. I needed to know this wasn't the end for us, that we could move on again, that we still had hope. In the midst of our grieving I badly needed to know. I needed hope. We needed hope to keep going and to help us get through. When I did get to talk to Dr Guerin, and he confirmed we could try again, I think it was what saved us, me for certain.

And so it was, a few months later, we started the process all over again. We still had four remaining pre-embryos frozen, so we went through the process of two more cycles, transferring two pre-embryos each time. We experienced the same excited expectation and hopefulness each time, but it all ended in disappointment. We didn't get pregnant again. When we had no more pre-embryos left, we wondered 'what now' again.

What were we to do? Give up? Giving up or throwing in the towel is not in our make-up, so the whole process started again: finding an egg donor, semen samples, tests and transfers. Maybe more disappointments would follow, but maybe not. If we succeeded, it would be worth it all. Starting this last cycle of IVF was also when we decided to go down the adoption route.

We travelled to Spain as before for the next IVF cycle. This time around we had four pre-embryos and as before we transferred two pre-embryos on two separate cycles. I never got pregnant again. We were at the stage when we had to give up. We didn't have a choice. I was now fifty and over the age of acceptance at the clinic.

10

ADOPTION

I get angry just thinking about the time we wasted on adoption. Thankfully we realised earlier than most that it was never going to happen for us, that we would never get a baby going this route. We had thought about adoption more and more as we experienced each failure with IVF. At least I did, maybe a lot more so initially than Seán, whereas surrogacy was something Seán had raised quite early on, even as we were first considering IVF. After IVF we agreed to go for adoption because it seemed, to me anyway, to be an easier, more straightforward process than surrogacy. I say that now, with tongue in cheek, having gone at least partway through that nightmare, they can only *claim* to be a process. Unfortunately for us, every aspect of our experience with the adoption process was a very unpleasant and bureaucratic one. Adoption was not and is not an option in Ireland today. Unfortunately, instead of being told this, instead of being honest with us and all the others out there still hoping, they encouraged us to get our hopes up. They led us to believe that we would get a baby, and so we spent time, precious time, going down this route.

We were one of the fortunate couples: we realised quickly we were getting nowhere and that we would never get the baby we desired through adoption. Of course, many wouldn't call two years in a process, 'quickly'. When we first applied to adopt, we waited almost twelve months to be called to what was described as an information meeting in Limerick. We couldn't figure out and we still can't understand why we had to wait so long to be called to a simple information meeting. It was in July during the busiest week for the pub trade in Miltown Malbay, but we traipsed along to a room in Limerick to join other couples and some solo applicants all in the same boat and on the same mission. There were two social workers in attendance and they addressed a room of approximately thirty people. They started by explaining what the assessment process entailed. The first bit of startling news was that because we were not married we actually could not apply as a couple. Instead, I would have to apply as a solo applicant. However, we would have to be jointly assessed, as Seán and I lived together. I remember wondering what bloody century we were living in. Why did we need to be married? Was it not possible for two unmarried people to adopt jointly? We couldn't apply together to adopt but we had to be assessed together? It was utter madness. Where did that leave a child who could be adopted by me but left Seán as the father with no legal rights? How was that good for a child?

They went on … should we still wish to pursue adoption after this meeting we would need to formally apply. I thought we had. But no, we would need to write in again formally requesting to be placed on the list for assessment. While we waited for the assessment to come through, we would be required to undergo a series of written assessments – homework for all intents and purposes.

Many questions were asked of the social workers, but they could only answer questions pertaining to the Health Service Executive (HSE) process itself. They couldn't even tell us what countries were open to Ireland for adoption. They actually couldn't tell us anything beyond the process of getting a declaration to adopt from the HSE. It was frustrating for us and it was evident that others in the room were feeling the same. The HSE seemed to be operating in a vacuum and in complete isolation of what was going on internationally in relation to adoption. Any questions that were asked outside of the assessment process went unanswered; they didn't know. It beggared belief and provided little hope that someday we might be parents. Unbelievably some of the hopeful parents-to-be in attendance were able to provide more information than the 'experts' themselves. Pushing our anger and frustration aside, we focused on why we were there. We were there for a reason and we were desperate for that reason to become a reality. We were all desperate in that room.

Following that meeting, we nonetheless applied formally and ended up completing the plethora of forms which would see us placed on the waiting list for assessment. We were still undergoing the last IVF cycle in Barcelona at that time but didn't dare mention it because during the meeting this was a question that was asked: what if you became pregnant during the process or what if you were going through IVF? The HSE were clear on that one. You would not be allowed to proceed any further with the adoption process if you became pregnant and you were excluded from applying at all if you were going through IVF. We wondered why it was unacceptable to conceive or be going through IVF while at the same time be fortunate enough to get a baby through adoption. Sure wouldn't that be a miracle?

Several months passed and we heard nothing. We were now completely finished with the IVF treatments and there was still no sign of an assessment on the horizon. Almost a year after the information meeting and about to give up, we were finally invited to attend a pre-assessment parenting course. Despite being parents already, good parents, it was still a requirement to attend this course in order to be placed on the list for the now ever-elusive assessment itself. The course was in Ennis, one day per week for four weeks, which meant we both had to take time off work to attend. In preparation, we completed all the documentation asked of us, spending hours and hours researching, preparing and completing cumbersome and lengthy written assignments, family trees, life-event charts, Garda clearance forms and reference forms. Everything we were asked to do, we did it.

Seán was up a pole doing a changeover when he received the call from one of the social workers requesting he attend a meeting in Limerick to discuss what they termed a 'very serious issue'. Worse again they told us this could affect us attending the course. We hadn't a clue what it was about, and they would not give us any inkling over the phone. According to them, the issue was too serious to be discussed over the phone. I panicked.

What if we were not allowed to attend, would we wait another year? Taking precious time off work, Seán went off to the meeting to be what he termed 'interrogated'.

It started by Seán being asked if he was sure he had been truthful about not having any convictions. This was in relation to his Garda clearance. 'Was there anything he wanted to tell them?' 'Did he need to think about his answer?' The clear insinuation was that he had lied on the Garda clearance form. 'You do have a conviction,' they told him. For the life of him Seán couldn't recollect any conviction against him, but it would seem he did have one which he omitted to tell them about. A number of years previously the pub had been the subject of a Gardaí visit over the Christmas period. The young lad working behind the bar had some customers on the premises after hours and as a consequence Seán, as the proprietor, received the summons. The fine was paid but it was recorded as a conviction and one which Seán had genuinely overlooked. Was it the oversight in not telling them about the conviction or was it the fact that he had a conviction that the social workers considered to be an extremely serious issue? It was obviously serious enough to require Seán to present himself in person to respond and equally serious enough that we might not be allowed to go any further in the adoption process. Seán was livid.

There were about nine other couples along with us, all naively hoping that this was the answer to our hopes and dreams of having a family. At this early stage we found ourselves having to choose the country we wanted to adopt from. We had to do our own research to find out what countries were open and available to Ireland to adopt from. This information was not forthcoming from the HSE. Vietnam was open and as we hadn't much choice,

Vietnam it was. Despite our reservations and probably, if we were honest, our annoyance at having to do a course such as this, it was surprisingly very interesting. It gave us a lot of insight into the psychology of adopting and the dos and don'ts of bringing a new baby home. The best part was all the interaction, discussion and networking amongst the group, while the most disappointing aspect was not being able to get up-to-date, relevant information on inter-country adoption. Information was again limited and only up to the point where one might be lucky enough to get a declaration from the HSE. Any other questions outside of this still couldn't be answered. Relevant questions such as where one could adopt from, what countries were open to us or what fees agencies charged remained frustratingly unanswered. Surely this basic information was sought out by every potential parent at these courses? So why wasn't the HSE prepared with answers? What we were able to glean from other people in the group was that we were very limited in what countries we would be able to go to for adoption. It seemed that since Ireland ratified the Hague Convention, countries were closing their doors to Ireland as opposed to opening them. Since then the only countries that Ireland could adopt from were those countries that had also ratified the Hague Convention or from Non-Hague countries with which Ireland had a bi-lateral agreement but unfortunately Ireland did not have any such agreements in place.

When and if we completed the assessment successfully a report, compiled by the social worker with her recommendation as to whether we should or should not be approved for adoption, would be sent to the Adoption Authority of Ireland for their final decision. If they approved us then we would receive our declaration allowing us to move to the next stage and adopt. The declaration would be valid for two years and if we had not managed to adopt within that period of time we might be able to get an extension or the application process would have to be gone through again. More significantly for us though was that if we proceeded now through the process we would not get a declaration for at least another five, six or even seven years. By which time because of our age we definitely would not be eligible to get a baby. We were told that we could get a child of seven or eight years old, maybe even older, and quite possibly we would be offered a child with special needs. As Seán's son Tomás has special needs we knew exactly what that entailed. It seemed that the HSE were deciding our destiny and our future, not us. Blinded to the reality by our desire to have a baby together we ploughed on thinking that maybe the process would change, maybe more countries would open up or the system might improve.

There were many strange moments during our experience with the Irish adoption 'process', but one in particular stands out. A surreal exercise during the course was each couple having to prepare a dish from their chosen country to share with the other participants. Was there a benefit to this exercise that we couldn't see with the exception of gorging on delicious food prepared at length on an evening following a long hard day at work?

Is adoption a realistic option for anyone in Ireland? We were another year on and no word or sign of an assessment. At that stage I think we were beginning to realise that adoption was not going to work for us. We moved on and left adoption behind us, in our heads anyway, while the HSE left us behind as we never heard another word from them. If we hadn't moved on would we have ever heard from them again? I doubt it somehow. Others whom we met at the course and who were further along in that journey were not as lucky as us to realise at an early enough stage that adoption was never going to happen. Many have ploughed on for as long as seven and eight years ever hopeful. During our time in the process we always heard, 'when you get your baby', never 'if' or 'maybe'. That was incredibly unfair. It is so wrong to manipulate people's emotions, to build up people's hopes and to allow them to think that they will get a baby, when in reality nothing is further from the truth.

Over the years we have met many people that gave so much: going through a lengthy interrogatory process; finally getting the declaration only to find that no countries were open to adopt from, and in the end, when their declarations had run out, they were either too old or too downtrodden and battle weary to go through it all again. In the end it was all for nothing; they didn't get a baby. We can't imagine the sadness and anger those people must feel seeing their hopes and dreams reduced to a glimmer and then to fade away altogether. It's not right, moral or fair to put people through that.

I remember getting a phone call a long time after from a couple who had been in our pre-assessment course with us. I couldn't believe they were still waiting. Their hope was waning and despair of ever getting a baby was creeping closer. Could we give them any advice? Yes, we could. Get out now!

Another day I was listening to an interview on the radio while driving. It was about a guy who did charitable work abroad in poor, under-developed and war-torn countries. He spoke about the children he came across scavenging for anything edible in the vastly increasing rubbish mountains. He described one little boy he had come across who was wearing a dirty old Nike sweatshirt. There was a red stain down the front, and as he was talking to the boy he began to suspect the stain was blood. Looking under the sweatshirt, he saw that part of the boy's bowel or large intestine was exposed. It was a congenital condition and there from birth. The rubbing and friction of the sweatshirt against his bowel was causing the bleeding. Apparently he was consensually orphaned, a child alone in the world. His mother had died and his father had remarried. Unfortunately, his father's new wife did not want him, so he had been forced to leave his home. This man, through the charity he worked for, was able to arrange for the boy to be brought to a hospital in Europe for corrective surgery, a relatively simple procedure. However, that little boy would at some stage have to return home to his country, return once again to scavenge amongst the discarded rubbish of millions. What was so sad and infuriating about this was that there were so many genuine people out there, like us, who would have given their eye teeth to take home and love this little boy as their own. But that would never happen.

11

SURROGACY

I suppose I dismissed surrogacy when Seán had raised it for a couple of reasons. Firstly, I was really convinced IVF would work for us. I wanted so much to have our baby. Secondly, there was almost an aura of illegality around the topic of surrogacy. This was borne out by the fact that we could not readily access information nor was it a topic of comfortable dinner-table conversation. In reality, this generally dissuades people from considering it as an option.

Following the failures of IVF and encouraged by Seán, I started researching surrogacy in the middle of 2012. My first port of call was to contact the fertility clinic we had attended in Ireland. I wanted some advice and enough information to allow us to make informed decisions. We naively presumed that in Ireland it was everyone's right to be able to access information and advice. However, the clinic wouldn't and couldn't speak to us because surrogacy is not permitted in Ireland. As there is no legislation governing surrogacy, it is therefore neither legal nor illegal and on that basis no information can be provided.

I must have contacted almost all of the fertility clinics in the country receiving the same response time and again. Once they heard I was enquiring about surrogacy they were unable to help or advise us. All gave that same reason. We found this difficult to understand. Why if surrogacy is not illegal could information not be provided on that basis and then let people as adults make up their own minds as to whether they wanted to avail of surrogacy or not?

The clinic in Barcelona was more forthcoming despite surrogacy not being permitted in Spain either. We were given details of websites to check out and a clinic in the USA was recommended to us, but it was also stressed that the costs involved were very high. The advice to us was to 'just let it go', mind you that was after we paid out a lot of money to this clinic without success.

With no other option and like a dog with a bone, I started researching online. Entering the word 'surrogacy' and hitting 'enter' produced an abundance of information. There were forums where people spoke of their own personal experiences with the various clinics abroad. The clinics had lots of online advertising. There were many websites, dedicated to sharing information, set up by people who had gone through surrogacy and were willing to help others. There were also other websites set up by organisations which appeared to operate independently of any clinic. The worst thing about researching online is trying to decipher what is factual, honest and accurate and what is just a PR exercise, out-of-date information or just plain old rubbish. I kept a journal to record relevant notes and material as I researched, keeping track of specific criteria and fees for each of the clinics. I didn't join any of the forums but I read them all, meticulously noting people's personal experiences and recommendations. People spoke openly of their successes and failures for all and sundry to read. I read it all avidly and could even empathise with some accounts of their failures. Clinical information such as success rates, waiting times, details of the process as well as the financial costs were available on most of the clinic websites with the eligibility criteria and costs varying greatly from country to country. There was also a plethora of middlemen and agencies out there willing to act on one's behalf, offering to help navigate the person through the process. Their promise was to ensure the person was treated fairly and not ripped off, but were they really necessary and worth the additional costs? Or were they the ones that might rip us off? We just didn't know.

We hit on a few websites, such as globaldoctoroptions.com, which were genuinely independent and objective and provided some really good detailed information. They are a not-for-profit organisation with the intention of ensuring all information is made available so that people can make informed decisions. This website provided a general overview of surrogacy in many countries with no requirement to subscribe.

Another website we stumbled upon was OneinSix.com set up by a couple from Australia who had attempted surrogacy ten times in India and had two successful pregnancies as a result. They popped up on lots of forums and websites wherever surrogacy was mentioned. They were advocating India as a destination for surrogacy, and while they provided lots of good information they were also putting themselves forward as agents able to negotiate with the clinics and help people navigate the whole process for a fee. If we hired them we would have to pay for their flights, accommodation and expenses, but again we wondered if we could trust them and if we needed them. While most of their information was of a practical nature – such as where to stay, what to eat and how to get from A to B – we later found out to our cost it was not always as accurate as one would have hoped. They invited interested people to email them with any queries or concerns which we did at the time and they generally responded very promptly. They were very upbeat about surrogacy and its success but at times almost too positive and pushy. Additional websites we found worth visiting were surrogacy.org.uk and www.surrogacy.com. Once my initial research was complete, I emailed and made contact with all the clinics on my list to get more detailed information from them about the process, costs and the law or regulations in relation to surrogacy in each respective country.

UKRAINE

Gestational surrogacy is legal in the Ukraine. Close enough to us in Ireland, flying time would be relatively short and it would be easy for us to travel over and back. The egg donor would be Caucasian, which might present us with fewer difficulties in the future. Clinics such as ISIDA, La Vita Felica or IRTSA were regulated and operated to specific criteria.

However, one of the eligibility criteria was that we had to be married for at least two years, so that ruled us out immediately. Despite being regulated, the cost of treatment varied greatly between clinics, ranging from €15,000 to €26,000 with additional costs of flights and accommodation. In the Ukraine, if one of the intending parents had a genetic link to the baby then the couple automatically had parental rights, but obviously that right did not transfer to Ireland. Also a surrogate mother could not refuse to hand the baby over to the intending parents, as surrogate mothers have no parental rights under Ukrainian law. Our initial communication with a clinic in the Ukraine did not raise our marital status as an issue. Later on, following my own research, I queried this, and it was confirmed as a criterion of the legislation in that country. At that point we moved on to look elsewhere. However, some time later the clinic made contact to ask if we still wanted to go ahead with surrogacy. I explained that we didn't meet the legislative criterion because we weren't married and so we couldn't go forward. The clinic then indicated without going into any detail that there could be a way around this requirement. We were a bit uncomfortable with this suggestion and knew we would have enough difficulties with the Irish law without entangling ourselves with other potential issues. It was a blessing really because had we proceeded we would have been right in the middle of a surrogacy process when all the political unrest erupted.

CYPRUS

I had been to Cyprus a few times in my life. I also had a very good friend from Cyprus who I knew would help us if we needed information or decided to go there for surrogacy. It is about a four-hour flight and an appealing country. However, there was very little information available on the internet, which seemed to indicate that not many people went there for surrogacy or there was deliberate secrecy around surrogacy in Cyprus for whatever reason. The clinic websites also had very little information. On a more positive note, the clinics were regulated, so we knew they had to conform to specific legislative criteria in order to operate.

We asked the same general questions of all the clinics, such as success rates, take-home rates, donor selection and costs. We expected that our questions would be answered readily and easily enough, but when we emailed a clinic in Cyprus they weren't as forthcoming with the information as one would have expected. My friend then checked out the clinic to see if she could get any more information for us. She quickly informed us that while the clinic was reputable, she still had difficulty getting some of the information for us. We had reservations as a result. What determined the clinic to be 'reputable' if we couldn't even get information? Unsubstantiated reports weren't enough.

USA

Surrogacy is legal in a number of states in the US. Consequently, there were a number of clinics available to us, for example, Circle Clinic, the Fertility Institute and Growing Generations. One major benefit for us in having a baby through surrogacy in the US was the entitlement to a US passport. This meant we could travel home easily and we could apply for an Irish passport for our baby on the basis of him or her holding a US passport. However, we would still face the same legal issues under Irish law once back home in Ireland.

We checked the clinic that was recommended to us and noted that it guaranteed a successful pregnancy. What this appeared to mean was that if we were unsuccessful in getting pregnant the first time, we could try again at no additional cost. While we wouldn't have to pay the clinic, we would still have additional costs of flights, accommodation and car hire.

However, the fees which ranged from €140,000 to €180,000 were cost prohibitive to us, no matter how much they guaranteed success. We just didn't have that funding at our disposal.

GREECE

In Greece, gestational altruistic surrogacy is legal and all other forms of surrogacy are illegal. There are specific legislative criteria to be met and permission for surrogacy to go ahead could only be granted by a court in Greece. Costs were in the region of €15,000 which was affordable for us, but the upper age limit for the intending mother was set at fifty years so we were ruled out on that basis alone.

UK

The UK allows gestational surrogacy while all other forms are illegal. Surrogacy is permissible for altruistic purposes as opposed to commercial purposes. However, it is legal only for couples residing in the UK.

INDIA

India is a main destination for surrogacy. In India, surrogacy is reportedly to be worth $1billion a year to the economy. Surrogacy in India has become increasingly popular for intending parents because costs are not prohibitive and in general the criteria for eligibility can be met. There are thousands of clinics offering IVF and surrogacy services operating in India. Importantly, while there is no legislation, the government has guidelines in place. Not all, but some of the clinics are regulated and operate within these guidelines and regulations. India has an Assisted Reproductive Technology Bill ready to be introduced into legislation aiming to regulate the surrogacy business, but changes in India's legislation can be a long and very protracted process. It is expected that this bill will increase the public's confidence in clinics by weeding out the dubious practitioners. In the meantime, we know there are many regulated and reputable clinics offering surrogacy services such as the Rotunda and the Corion in Mumbai, the Akanksha clinic in Anand and Delhi IVF in New Delhi. Costs are approximately €15,000 to €20,000 depending on the treatment plan required, then add to that the flights and accommodation. There will be additional costs no matter what country is chosen; these include DNA testing, legal costs and hospital costs. For Irish people the increasing legal costs to deal with the Irish legal system on return to Ireland is another bitter but necessary pill to swallow. To put it further into perspective, surrogacy in India is about one third of the cost of surrogacy in the UK.

12

CHOOSING A CLINIC

There are thousands of clinics operating in India. Not all are regulated and this was an essential factor for us when it came to choosing the clinic. Overall the feedback on the various online forums was positive, particularly on clinics like the Rotunda, Corion, Akanksha and Delhi IVF, and the testimonials on these clinics' websites also proved very positive. Mumbai appealed to us as a place in India to go to, as it is less crowded than Delhi and is considered more sophisticated and modern than Anand.

The next step was to email both the Rotunda and the Corion clinics with our long list of questions, which included:

- What was their overall success rate for donor egg surrogacy?
- How many trips would we need to make to India?
- How much would the total cost be?
- What was the 'take home' baby success rate?
- How long would we have to remain in India for?
- Would both our names be on the birth certificate?
- How could we optimise our chances of having a baby?
- Was there any way we could optimise our chances of having twins? For example, was it an option to have two surrogate mothers?

While we had some information on the various clinics in India, we didn't have enough, and we didn't know anyone who had gone through surrogacy in any country let alone India. We still knew too little of the overall process. Response from both clinics was swift. The Rotunda was founded in 1963 so was very well established. It had a good success rate, however, it was a possibility that we would have to go on a waiting list due to demand for egg donors and surrogates at the clinic. The Corion Clinic on the other hand was only established in 2010 under the direction of Dr Kushal Kadam. While the clinic was new and still only establishing itself as a player in this field, Dr Kadam, the clinical director, had worked previously in the Rotunda where she was the medical director and main point of contact for intending couples. Success rates were good and, importantly for us, there was no waiting time if we chose to go with an Indian egg donor as opposed to a Caucasian egg donor. Ironically, if we wanted a Caucasian egg donor those eggs would generally be retrieved from a Ukrainian donor. In the overall scheme of things, whether the donor was Caucasian or Indian didn't matter a whit to us, and we were happy to go with an Indian egg donor, particularly when the waiting time was less.

The Corion Clinic was already ticking all the boxes for us, so we went ahead and checked the list of global ambassadors on their website. Global ambassadors are generally people who have successfully gone through the process in that clinic and allow their names and contact details to be listed on the website for other intending parents to make contact. There was no listing for Ireland, but there was one couple from the UK and another couple from Australia listed. Both couples responded to our emails and were very positive about the clinic, the overall service and Dr Kadam. The clinic answered all our queries and sent us a schedule of fees which outlined all the payment stages. The total cost for our particular needs would come to Rs. 1,380,000 which was about €19,422. We would pay more if our surrogate was to carry twins. The cost of the delivery and care for our surrogate while in hospital would also be extra, about €1,500. If there were any complications or if neonatal care was required, the costs would increase again. In addition, we would also have the legal fees in India. Based on the information we got from the various sources, the fact that the Corion Clinic was regulated and conformed to all government guidelines, the costs involved were manageable and there was no wait time, we decided on the Corion Clinic in Mumbai as our destination.

Decision made, we contacted Dr Kadam to commence the process as soon as possible. We first had to satisfy Dr Kadam that we were medically suitable candidates for surrogacy and that we met the clinic's criteria for inclusion on the programme. We had to provide evidence that we were unable to have children by natural means and that we had undergone treatment to no avail. We emailed as much of the documentation as possible regarding our attempts at IVF and posted on what couldn't be emailed. We would have to repeat some of the tests again because of the lapse of time, but we were accepted onto the programme and could commence the process immediately. With the registration forms completed, we were ready to rock.

Because Seán would be the biological father, he was obliged to have a number of tests carried out. Some were the usual blood tests while others were genetic tests to rule out any unforeseen complications or difficulties. All were very similar to the tests already undertaken for our treatments in Barcelona.

A copy of the contract landed in the post, which we had to complete and return to the clinic. We would receive the original contract fully completed and signed by all parties – the clinic, the surrogate mother and ourselves – when we attended the clinic for our first visit. The contract was very lengthy and was written in legal terminology, which made it difficult to understand fully. At this point we contemplated getting legal advice but decided not to once we read over it a few times. Following a little effort and deciphering, it became obvious that there wasn't anything contentious in it that warranted a legal opinion.

There was one section which caused us some anxiety and worry but not from a legal perspective. We had to appoint one or two people who would assume responsibility for our unborn baby if both of us were to die before the baby was born. We had told no one about our plans so how could we ask anyone to do this and even if we had told people could we put such an enormous responsibility on someone? We knew the risk of us both dying was minimal but nevertheless it prompted us to think, what if? We couldn't complete this section of the contract, so we just left it blank for the time being anyway. We felt we could always go back to it if we got pregnant.

13

DONORS & DONATION

A few days later we got a number of egg-donor profiles, eight in total. We were also told that if we didn't find an acceptable donor from this list, we could request additional profiles. Each profile was set out on an A4 page along with a photograph and details such as the donor's name, age, religion, education, colour, marital status, number of pregnancies and whether the births were normal or not, along with the delivery type, number and ages of children. Also included were details of any illness the donor, her children, siblings or parents had, as well as a comprehensive hormone profile. We ended up with even more questions after going through the profiles, as we didn't understand some of the information. For example, we didn't understand the education grading system and some of the medical terms in the profiles. While we weren't that concerned with the educational grading system we wanted to understand everything before making a decision.

We knew what the optimum age for an egg donor should be and what the hormone levels should be. Once we had a handle on all the information, we separately chose three profiles each. What was notable was that we both picked two of the same donors. Seán's interest was really focused on medical history and whether the donor or her family had any illnesses, while for me it was the age and the hormone levels that were important. I felt these were good indicators as to how likely the donor would be in providing a good number of healthy viable eggs. By a process of discussion and elimination we eventually whittled our choice down to one donor who we were both happy to go with. Just before Christmas 2012, we sent our decision to Dr Kadam. Mrs KIS was our chosen donor. Unfortunately, due to 'family issues', Mrs KIS was no longer available as an egg donor. Maybe it was fate or all for luck that we had to go back and choose again. So, it was on Christmas Eve 2012 our donor was finally chosen – Mrs MSH.

According to Dr Kadam, Mrs MSH's treatment in preparation for harvesting the eggs was to begin immediately. We wondered if Seán's sample could be taken in a clinic in Ireland and transported to India. We considered this to cut costs for us. The clinic agreed that it could be done. Apparently people in other countries but not Ireland had already done this, so it wasn't new to them.

We were the first Irish couple to attend the Corion Clinic for surrogacy. There was a single person from Ireland who had attended the Corion a few months previously and was now successfully pregnant. We thought that person was so brave to be undertaking such a journey alone. On hindsight we really didn't realise how brave that person actually was. We presumed we could attend a clinic in Ireland where Seán would give the sample, and the Corion Clinic would then arrange for the sample to be transported to India. So we set about sourcing a clinic which would take the sample, store it and release it to the transport service. It couldn't be such a difficult task.

We hit a brick wall, as none of the clinics in Ireland would take a semen sample for the purposes of surrogacy. We phoned the clinics and explained to them what we needed. We reiterated to each clinic that we only wanted the sample to be taken, held and released to a transport service. It didn't matter, they wouldn't do it. We then contacted the clinic in Spain to see if they could do it, however, they couldn't help us either; they were limited to giving us advice and information only.

Searching closer to home again, we looked towards London and clinics such as Andrology Solutions, the Assisted Reproduction and Gynaecology Centre and the Assisted Conception Unit. We contacted one in particular which was recommended by Dr Kadam, the Centre for Reproductive and Genetic Health (CRGH). While they were willing to take the samples for transportation they had to first check with the Human Fertilisation and Embryology Authority (HFEA) that they were permitted to do so. The HFEA act as the UK regulator of IVF treatment and research involving human pre-embryos, and they license and monitor UK fertility clinics. While they do allow the retrieval of semen samples for the purpose of transportation outside the country, there is a requirement for the receiving centre to meet a number of legislative criteria as set out in the General Directions 0006 – Import and Export of Gametes and Pre-embryos, Schedule 4 (General Directions).

Both the CRGH and I contacted the Corion Clinic requesting they provide the proof necessary to show that they met the required General Directions. In turn, Dr Kadam provided the clinic's credentials, namely that the clinic met all of the General Directions legislative criteria, that their certification was ISO 9001:2008. They were also registered with the Indian Council of Medical Research (ICMR) and accredited by the Indian Society of Assisted Reproduction (ISAR). But all that wasn't enough and what followed was a plethora of emails back and forth between the clinic, the HFEA and us. The CRGH said in one correspondence to us that they felt that because of the 'nature of the treatment' the clinic in India was 'unlikely to meet' the General Directions. It was a vague and ambiguous response, and we couldn't figure out what it meant. It was Dr Kadam's clear opinion that her clinic did conform to the General Directions, but it was also her opinion that because the 'nature of the treatment' that was being referred to in the correspondence was surrogacy it would be unacceptable in any event for the HFEA to cooperate or work with the Corion Clinic. Without specifying the reasons why, the overall response from the HFEA was that the clinic did not conform.

The CRGH did, however, state that we could submit an application to the HFEA detailing our specific circumstances, and our case would be considered on an individual basis. There was no time frame given for a decision on this, and also, in the unlikely event of being accepted, there were costs involved. A consultation fee and the cost of retrieving and freezing the sample would be in the region of £1,000. Then we needed to add on the cost of hotels and flights to the UK. It was beginning to look like a more expensive option than going directly to India. Of more serious concern to us was that the sample would have to be held in quarantine in the UK for six months. This was too long for us. It was time we didn't have. While the clinic had endeavoured to meet the criteria of the HFEA in order to facilitate us, we were increasingly frustrated with the obstacles presented at every juncture. We had lost enough time; we were going to India.

What we didn't know at the time was that this first trip to India was in fact one of the best decisions we made. It gave us an insight into life in India as well as an opportunity to check out the hospital and other hotel accommodation. This ensured it wouldn't be near as daunting if we were ever lucky enough to return.

14

BELOW THE RADAR

Sometime in September 2012, Below the Radar, a TV production company working on a documentary about Irish couples and surrogacy, contacted us to ask if we would be willing to participate. During their research for the documentary they had come across the Aussie couple on the various forums and websites and had made contact with them. As they were looking specifically for Irish couples, the Aussies had given them our contact details.

Communication was initially by email, followed by a telephone conversation with the producer. We considered participating but thought maybe we could do so anonymously, as we were not interested in going public at any stage about our efforts. Most importantly, we didn't know where this journey would lead us. We might be successful, we might not be successful, but if we were, then we had to think of our baby in all of this. Denise, the producer, was persistent to say the least and asked to meet with us. In October 2012, on a dark miserably wet night, we met with her and her colleague, Nicole, in a local hotel. We sat well away from other people towards the front of the hotel, not wishing anyone to hear our whispered conversation. We were terrified that we would be overheard.

We gave them an account of where we were at in the surrogacy process, and they in turn outlined what their intentions were in making the documentary. They were a company commissioned by RTÉ to make the documentary on surrogacy from an Irish perspective and as such were seeking Irish people who would agree to participating. Remaining anonymous was ruled out very quickly. If we agreed to participate, the plan was to follow and film our journey for the duration, whatever the outcome might be. We couldn't agree. We felt we were embarking on too difficult and too personal a journey. We knew there would be some people who would not approve of our course of action in realising a family together and who would judge us as being wrong for whatever their reasons. But we weren't unduly concerned about those people. We were more worried about the impact of going public would have on our child if we were successful in our endeavours. There had to be others out there willing to participate in their documentary, but apparently there were no couples willing to go public on the subject. Even though we felt we didn't need the additional pressure of the documentary being made about us, Denise presented a strong case. They highlighted some very crucial points, for example, if surrogacy continued to be something that was brushed under the carpet in Ireland, it would never be recognised in law in this country. Children, like ours, born through surrogacy would continue to be non-existent in the eyes of our legislators and government. They left soon after but not before sowing the seed of doubt in our subconscious and asking us to consider their proposal over the coming weeks. They would contact us after Christmas. If we were still opposed to participating, they would graciously accept that.

Denise had mentioned a conference on surrogacy being held in University College Cork in November. Conferences on surrogacy didn't arise too frequently in Ireland, so in the hope that I would get some information of benefit I went along. It was open to the public but appeared to be more focused on the legal aspects, as many of the presenters were from a legal background and most of the attendees were college law students. Despite this, it was extremely informative, giving a clear outline of the process of surrogacy as well as highlighting other issues we hadn't considered around equality, the legislation and children's rights. It mentioned the international perspective but focused particularly on the UK and significantly, it was the first time that I heard mention of the guidelines for Irish people entering into surrogacy arrangements abroad. This document entitled, 'Citizenship, Parentage, Guardianship and Travel Document Issues in Relation to Children Born as a Result of Surrogacy Arrangements Entered into Outside the State' (Irish Surrogacy Guidelines) set out what we had to comply with in order to be able to return home with a baby born through surrogacy abroad. In stark contradiction, the government had these guidelines in place, a clear acknowledgement that surrogacy is happening, yet they will not provide or allow for the provision of information to couples seeking these services. I remember thinking it was a pity there wasn't more of these conferences held, because they do help those desperately seeking information as well as educating those who remain ignorant on the subject.

Our last Christmas before embarking on our journey came and went quietly. We were excited about the prospect of having a family together but also quietly fearful of failure again. At times we spoke about the documentary and discussed the pros and cons of participating. Why would we put ourselves out there in the public eye? Why would we expose ourselves to criticism and judgement, leaving ourselves even more vulnerable than we already were? Wouldn't going public make things difficult, maybe impossible, for a child of ours in years to come? We live in Catholic Ireland and people have views and opinions entrenched in Catholicism. Wouldn't this give rise to harsh judgement? We thought too of the difficult road we had already walked – the IVF, the pain of losing a baby – and now the excitement of thinking that maybe this option, this very last option might actually work. We knew of some couples who were struggling to start a family and wondered about those couples: would they ever contemplate or even think of surrogacy as an option if we didn't present it as one? We thought of the struggle we had to get any information in Ireland and we again wondered why do we, as a nation, still accept that we have no right to access information? Don't we have a right to make up our own minds? Don't we have a right to make our own decisions that affect our lives? Why do we continue to allow our government to sweep these issues under the carpet or export them abroad? We had no answers and it was this fact that finally prompted our decision to participate in the documentary. We wanted to put surrogacy out there as an option for people. We wanted to give them information and an insight into the process of surrogacy. After that, whether people chose to go that route or not would be entirely their own decision. Importantly, it would be their decision and no one else's. And maybe just maybe, in time, by pushing the issue into the public realms for discussion, we might influence the government into introducing legislation.

The phone rang early one January morning in 2013. I could hear the anxiety in Denise's voice as she asked if we had made the decision. Maybe it was the end of the road for their documentary if we refused. But I said, 'yes we have and yes we will'. I could hear the sharp intake of breath while I ploughed on to explain our reasons for doing so. As she spoke, it was obvious that she was both relieved and excited to have found a couple willing to go public with this subject. We talked for some time discussing practicalities such as organising the initial interviews. I have a sneaking feeling Denise may have also been a little worried that we might change our minds, and she intended to get the ball rolling as quickly as possible just in case. The crew would travel to our home within the next week to commence filming, as the time frame was so short before making our first trip to India. And so it began; one thing we weren't sure of at that stage was how long the film crew would be a part of our lives.

15

PREPARING FOR INDIA

We needed to sort out accommodation for our week-long stay in Mumbai. Online research revealed an abundance of hotels and how expensive accommodation was there. The cheapest two- and three- star hotels cost up to €120 per night. We hadn't a clue which were good or bad and what areas to avoid. The clinic recommended using an agency called 'i World Tours' and Puneet was the gentleman tasked with sourcing accommodation for potential clients. Obviously it isn't a requirement to use an agency but we did for a number of reasons. We didn't know Mumbai and we had limited time available, therefore we knew we would feel more secure on this first trip having the expertise of someone on the inside. We only had a week in Mumbai to get everything sorted and we needed someone who could navigate us through the myriad of our requirements, someone who could quickly get things for us at short notice, such as a local SIM card. We were also thinking ahead. If we were to return later in the year, it might not be so bad to have someone local in our corner.

We told Puneet that we wanted a reasonably priced hotel close to the clinic and to restaurants and shops. He sent us a range of options and following a bit more online research we decided on the three-star Emerald Hotel and Apartments in Juhu. During my own search, I noted the price of this particular hotel was cheaper online than Puneet's estimate, so I pointed this out to him. He quickly reverted and apologetically offered us a lower price and also threw in two-way airport transfers. We were a bit dubious about him but still went ahead and booked through him. However, instead of paying before we travelled, we arranged to meet up upon arrival at the hotel to pay him directly. That was our safeguard.

For our trip to India we were required to have tourist visas, a straightforward enough process. Completing the application forms online, uploading the passport-size photos, printing off the forms and sending them to the Indian embassy in Dublin along with our passports was relatively simple. Within two weeks we had the passports and visas back in our hands and all seemed in order.

We were scheduled to fly to India on 30 January returning on 6 February. However, in mid-January, Dr Kadam emailed to say that they had started the stimulation of our donor, Mrs MSH, and she would more than likely be ready for egg retrieval on 27 or 28 January. We needed to be in India earlier than planned, so we changed the flights to 26 January with our return flight now on 2 February.

Now all that was left was to tell some people what we were up to before jetting off into the sunset. Just a couple of weeks before we were due to fly out, my brother Don was home for a few days, and we took the opportunity to tell him. His reaction was as expected: cool as you like, he just laughed at what he thought was absolute madness, but he was accepting in his own whatever-makes-you-happy outlook on life. Marion, Seán's sister, was next on the list and her reaction was also entirely as expected: 'Ah Jesus, why can't ye act yer age?' Last but not least was Donal. He reacted like everyone else: supportive and happy for us. Of course Noel and Ann were told not only for their friendship but Noel would be carrying the can at work while Seán was away. Once we had these few told we felt better. If anything happened to us while out there or en route at least a few people knew what we were up to. We would tell our remaining close circle of friends – Emer and Mike, Mary and Scruff, Mairéad and David, Máire and Tom and Breda and Tony – if we were fortunate enough to be making a return trip.

On Saturday, 26 January 2013, we began our journey to India. The small film crew of just Denise and Edel, the director, was shadowing us. We would travel together from Dublin Airport. While checking our visas, the steward noted a problem. Seán's name on his visa didn't match his passport because it was spelled incorrectly. She would have to check with her supervisor to see if the visa was acceptable to travel on or not. At that time, a section of the visa was handwritten, and it was this handwritten section that had misspelled Seán's name; they had spelled it Sián. I felt so stupid. I hadn't even noticed it before, as the writing was so small. The steward explained that while we might be able to travel out, there could be problems on the other side. Worst case scenario, we wouldn't be allowed to enter India.

She went off to check with her supervisor and panic set in. If we couldn't travel, we would lose this opportunity and have to start the process all over again, perhaps with another egg donor. Certainly it would mean another cycle and preparation process. I was in turmoil while Seán remained calm. The steward returned, granted us permission to fly but warned us of the possibility of problems at immigration on the other side. We didn't care, once we could go. We would deal with the problem then, if there was one.

Flight EK504 into Chhatrapati Shivaji International Airport (BOM) Mumbai was uneventful. We couldn't sleep with the terrifying excitement battling inside us. As we traversed the continents we must have watched about four films while Denise and Edel snored obliviously. Just before landing, we completed the obligatory immigration declarations and had our visas and passports at the ready when we joined the arduously slow and lengthy lines of weary travellers waiting to be scrutinised at immigration. Strict rules were in effect and the stern unsmiling immigration officials were going to ensure we all abided. Our visas, passports and declarations were checked, turned this way and that way, scrutinised while we held our breath. With this level of scrutiny the error could not be missed. Then just as suddenly, and with a wave of his hand … we were through.

16

INDIA

India reminds me of a Refresher, that childhood sweet, melting, bubbling and bursting into a myriad of fizzy sweet and sour flavours, frothing up in your mouth so that you had to suck in your cheeks, purse your lips together and squeeze your eyes closed. That is what India is: a kaleidoscope of colour, flavours, smells and vibrancy which infuses every part of your being. Seán had been to India over twenty years previously and while he probably remembered a little of what to expect, a lot had changed. Quite unexpectedly and almost instantaneously we both loved the country. Although we only saw a very minute part of India, what we saw only whetted our appetite for more. Irrespective, we knew we would return someday and we hoped that when that day came we would have our child with us to show him or her where they came from.

Mumbai, the capital of Maharashtra and formerly Bombay, is the most populated city in India with an estimated 18.4 million people. It is one of the most populated cities in the world and is also the wealthiest city in India with the highest number of billionaire and millionaire residents. In stark contrast, as we flew in low over Mumbai towards the runway, we could see below us the vastness of the Dharavi slum. Anyone who has watched the film *Slumdog Millionaire* will know that slums are a foundation of life in India and in particular Mumbai. Over 50 per cent of Mumbai's population live in slums and the largest slum not only in India but in the whole of Asia is Dharavi. It is home to over one million people – with factories and shops within this city in a city – all working, trading, selling and even more astonishingly, exporting goods. In fact, Mumbai's business opportunities, as well as its potential to offer a higher standard of living, attract migrants from all over India, making the city a melting pot of many communities and cultures.

But out on the streets of Mumbai deprivation is all encompassing. The squalor is immeasurable, the poverty immense. What is even harder to comprehend is how the impoverished, living on the streets, existing under bridges and in makeshift huts can reside in such benign acceptance amongst the very wealthy and affluent section of the population. In India, 70 per cent of the population live in poverty where people are homeless and simply exist day to day begging for money or food. They have nothing. They grapple daily to stay alive. The streets are crammed full of beggars, young and old, many with missing limbs or even eyes. Some have been cut off, removed or gouged out so they would get a more sympathetic response from the public while begging. Those unable to walk manoeuvred expertly but perilously on makeshift boards fitted with wheels in and out of the traffic. They tread silently from car to car tapping softly almost apologetically on windows, hoping for the window to open that tiny crack. Hands stretched out expectantly, ready to grasp whatever is thrown to them. All the begging, the desolation, the deprivation and serenity, the faces that had lived a thousand years in just ten, shocked us into speechlessness and a complete inability to even react. There were too many. We were overwhelmed.

Then there were the 'he/shes': a derogatory name but what they are known as in Mumbai. The transvestites are considered the lowest of the low, society's outcasts. They met in specific areas of the city, presumably because there was safety in numbers, plying their trade and begging like all the others. People in general ignored these misfortunes quite easily. The taxi drivers advised us never to open the windows and more importantly not to attempt to give money to anyone begging let alone the 'he/shes'. We grappled with this advice but soon understood after we gave money on a few occasions. Once you made any attempt to give money to someone you would find yourself immediately besieged by dozens more, emerging from the shadows pulling at your clothes, surrounding you, grasping for that elusive rupee. The taxi drivers, as a result, would become angry with us and their wrath was another thing we preferred not to experience more than once. Ignoring someone deliberately is not an easy thing to do, particularly when your conscious gnaws away at you. It was always a struggle to ignore the children; we wanted to help. Of course we wanted to give them money, but we were also aware that there were too many, too many small frail children, too many women carrying babies, men with no arms or legs, the old and the blind – all begging, begging for the right to survive. It was so constant and so in our faces all the time that it was something we found very hard to get our heads around and accept. We knew the only way and the best way was not to make eye contact with any of them.

In India the caste system determines social standing, caste being the basic social structure of Hindu society. There are a number of layers within the caste system, and it is believed that one is born into a caste depending on how one has lived in a previous life. For example, if a person has lived a good moral life then there is a chance of that person being reborn into a higher caste. This caste system imparts great influence in significant areas of life such as employment and marriage. What did these poor people think they did in a previous life to warrant living such a miserable existence in this life?

Mumbai is a city that never sleeps: traffic never stops, noise never ceases and people never stop partying. You will never want for any type of food in Mumbai: the most delicious vegetarian food; the most flavoursome rice and noodle dishes; the most exotic fish and the fieriest curries all add to a wonderful culinary experience. Street stalls sell the tastiest morsels of food that you eat from little bags made from very carefully wrapped old newspaper. The restaurants are always busy, the bars always full and nightclubs always teeming with young people all partying, every night of the week.

Shopping in India is also a delight, well for me it was anyway! Markets, centuries-old bazaars, vast modern westernised shopping malls and streets lined with stalls all fuse to sell a staggering array of goods. Someone said to us during our stay, 'You can get anything you want in India.' It was absolutely true. Imagine having a bespoke suit made to order in six hours. It's absolutely possible and Seán can testify to this. Then there were the street vendors: little old men and women squatting on their hunkers with a small set of weighting scales used to meticulously weigh their colourful aromatic spices and herbs whose names we couldn't pronounce let alone know what to do with. Stalls lined the streets teeming with perfectly ripened fruits and brightly coloured vegetables. We marvelled at how they could grow and harvest such a variety and amount of exotic produce from such a dry and barren land.

17

THE CORION CLINIC

Emerging from a hugely overcrowded, chaotic and disorganised airport into blistering heat was a serious shock to an Irish body unaccustomed to the sun. Mumbai's arid, dry and dusty heat would fry you in minutes. Our Irish eyes, unused to the sun, took a few minutes to adjust as we squinted around trying to locate our hotel transport. Arriving at our hotel we quickly checked in, deposited our bags and headed straight for the clinic. Our appointment was for 10.30 a.m. Tired, hot and sweating, we travelled across town to the clinic. I was becoming anxious because we were already late for the appointment. Nothing on earth prepares you for the nightmare of traffic in Mumbai. Beeping horns is incessant and sitting in traffic for hours is a pastime for all city goers.

Our taxi turned into a side street eventually and pulled up outside a large concrete building. It didn't look like a clinic. There were no signs and on even closer inspection we thought we had been brought to the wrong place. Seeing us hesitate prompted the taxi driver to wave us around towards the back of the building. He kept pointing and beckoning at us to go on. Moving in the general direction we saw steps leading up to a side entrance, and as we approached we noticed a small sign for the clinic on a wall inside the building. Our first impressions weren't great; this looked to be a far cry from the clinic we had attended in Barcelona. To say that it wasn't very inviting or pleasant looking was putting it mildly. The building looked very basic, almost unfinished, and it certainly didn't look like a place where clinical or medical procedures were carried out. Inside the entrance to the three-story building, the hallway was grubby and the stairs were a series of bare stone steps. The sign for the clinic pointed to the third floor, and as we headed up the stairs we passed many Indian women all sitting or standing around, giggling and chatting. As we ascended towards them, they retreated into a smiling silence, gazing and watching closely as we passed. Each and every one of them were dressed in the obligatory saris that were always vivid and colourful, beautifully accessorised with jewelled sandals and copious amounts of sparkling jewellery. We will never know, but perhaps one of those beautiful elegant ladies was our egg donor. Just outside the clinic door was a small annex housing boxes of disposable shoe covers. All visitors to the clinic were obliged to put on shoe covers before entering while staff were required to remove their shoes altogether and put on regulation clinic shoes.

Behind the reception desk just inside the door sat a number of staff. They overlooked the tiny waiting area which could seat about eight people in total. This area was dominated by a large flat-screen TV on the wall, which provided some diversion. A young man offered water or tea, a common custom in shops and offices throughout India. We realised we needn't have worried about being late for our appointment, as we were left watching TV for nearly another hour. During that time, while watching the comings and goings, we noticed that the area was refreshingly devoid of photo albums of smiling babies or glossy baby pictures adorning the walls. While the area we sat in was a shoebox in comparison to the waiting rooms we had occupied in Ireland and Spain, it was faultless and spotlessly clean.

The original contract was returned to us, this time signed by everyone involved. In one of our conversations with Dr Kadam before we had travelled to India we asked if we would be able to meet our egg donor. In India egg donors remain anonymous so we would not be allowed to meet her, however, she did say there was a chance we might see her in the clinic, as she may be there at the same time as us. I found myself looking at every Indian woman, wondering if it was her and unsure as to why I felt the need to see her in the first place. It was most likely to see what our child might look like.

Seán supplied his sample, after which we were called into Dr Kadam's office. It was again a small space but perfectly organised. Dr Kadam had been asked by Edel and Denise in advance of travelling for permission to film at the clinic to which she had no objection, so we all squeezed into the tiny room. There's nothing like being up close and personal.

We had our list of questions to hand so that we wouldn't forget anything, and we began by asking her the following:

- Would she outline the whole process again for us?
- Would Seán be required to give more than one sample?
- Were the eggs already harvested?
- When would we know how many eggs we had?
- When would we know how many pre-embryos we had?
- How many pre-embryos were recommended to transfer for an optimum chance of success?
- When would the transfer happen?
- When would we choose the surrogate mother?
- Would we actually meet the surrogate mother?
- Was there a surrogate house and if so could we visit the house?
- When would we know if our surrogate was pregnant?
- How would we be informed: email, phone call or Skype?
- If successful, would we be able to Skype our surrogate at a later stage from Ireland?
- If successful, would we get regular medical reports?
- What happened if we were unsuccessful?

We had so many questions to ask and Dr Kadam gave us her undivided attention. She was professional and clinical in answering all our questions. I jotted down the answers quickly so that we could read back over the information. There was such an awful lot to take in and assimilate.

It had already been explained to us that we would not be allowed to meet the donor because all egg donations must be anonymous, however, we were told we could ask our egg donor any questions via Dr Kadam. She also confirmed that we could not visit the surrogate house. The reason given for this was that the area where the house was located was residential, and if visiting were allowed it might attract attention from the locals and neighbours. Surrogacy it would seem was not an entirely acceptable practice in India, and the surrogate mothers did not relish unwelcome attention. Instead we were treated to photographs of the house shown to us from Dr Kadam's laptop. In response to our other questions, Dr Kadam told us we would be choosing the surrogate mother that day and also confirmed that they would be doing a day three embryo transfer.

As she worked through our list of questions, Dr Kadam also told us that there was legislation on surrogacy and assisted human reproduction pending in India, but that it had been pending for a long time and there was no indication as to when this legislation might be introduced. In the meantime, though, she said that the Indian government was in the process of introducing new visa rules entitled 'Change in Visa Guidelines for Intending Parents Wishing to Avail of Surrogacy Services in India' (Indian Visa Guidelines). This essentially would mean that people would have to apply for a medical visa as opposed to a tourist visa when travelling to India for surrogacy, and in order to be granted a medical visa, the applicants would need to comply with criteria contained within these Indian Visa Guidelines. A list of people's names would be sent by her to the Foreign Regional Registration Offices (FRRO), requesting that these people already in the surrogacy process be exempt from having to comply with the Indian Visa Guidelines; our names would be included in that list.

18

SHOBHA

Some of the women we had passed on the stairs came and went from the clinic. Other women emerged from rooms deep within the clinic to use the one shared toilet, all glancing, smiling shyly at us. The young man came to us several times with more offerings of water and tea. At the back of the clinic and across from Dr Kadam's office, we had passed two small areas screened off from the world by curtains. It was behind these curtains that many of the women retreated to. We weren't sure, but it looked like another waiting area, and whenever we looked in that direction, we could see the women peeping out at us, giggling and chattering away.

Quite unexpectedly, a group of six women emerged from the room, walked straight up to where we were sitting and stood in a line in front of us. Frozen, we sat and stared in this very small but busy and public waiting area while a staff member, one of the doctors at the clinic, handed us a sheaf of A4 papers and explained, in reasonably good English, that we were to choose our surrogate mother from this group. What she had handed us was their profiles. Quite taken aback, we looked at the women first and then read the profiles without really knowing where to start or what we should be looking for. We hadn't expected this. We weren't sure what we expected, but it wasn't to be choosing from a line-up of women in a public waiting room.

Information on the women's profiles was similar to the donor profiles, including physical and personal characteristics, health and family history, fertility history and investigations carried out. Again, it was difficult to understand some of the information so we asked the doctor to explain. We then asked which of the women was most prepared medically to receive a transfer. All the women were beautiful, some tall, some small, all smiling shyly at us, all waiting for their lives to change, all hoping to be picked. We wondered how many times they had lined up like this, to be accepted or rejected. Pointing to one profile the doctor indicated that this woman was best prepared. For that reason alone we choose our surrogate mother Shobha Dinesh Pandey.

With disappointment etched on their faces, the remaining women silently retreated into the room at the back of the clinic to sit and wait presumably for the next line-up in front of intending parents. Shobha was standing alone in front of us. She probably had no idea why we had chosen her above the others, but we smiled reassuringly at her. We asked her name but she remained impassive, staring blankly back at us until we realised she didn't speak English. We asked the same doctor again to translate for us and also if we could go somewhere more private to talk. We were shown into a small room with a single examination couch. No chairs or any other furniture could be accommodated in the tiny room. Shobha and I sat on the couch while Seán stood with the doctor. We asked Shobha if she was happy to be chosen as our surrogate, why she was doing this and what it meant for her and her family. Shobha replied very quietly and serenely, shaking her head from side to side ever so slightly as is the Indian custom. She was happy to do it because she would have money as a result to build a house and educate her children. She would be able to make a better life for her family, particularly her children. She had two boys aged seven and five. Shobha was beautiful, shy and gentle as she smiled and allowed us to take photos. Seán was emotional as he thanked her for what she was agreeing to do for us. It is an overwhelming concept to think that this woman was willing to give up nine months of her life to carry our baby. The sacrifice involved and Shobha's generosity could never be reciprocated.

We would need to return to the clinic on Wednesday, 30 January for the transfer. Only two days to kill. That afternoon was spent settling into the hotel, checking out the surrounding area and soaking up India: the smells, the heat, the noise and the whole atmosphere of this country. By the evening we were knackered so decided we would head out for dinner and get to bed early, so that we'd be in form for sightseeing the next day. Famous last words. We might have been knackered, but we were also on a high after the day. So while we went out early, we can't confess to going to bed early. We feasted on Indian fare and drank large wonderfully cold bottles of Kingfisher beer before returning to the hotel bar to wait for Puneet to arrive. While waiting we enjoyed more Kingfishers.

Puneet was a friendly young man. After we paid for our hotel, he joined us for a drink. We had a good long chat about the area, where to go to eat, the markets and shopping and the best places to go sightseeing. He offered to drive us around one of the days to show us the sights as well as to see other accommodation available if we were to return later in the year. This was definitely an offer we couldn't refuse. Puneet knew we could be future customers, and if we were satisfied with his service now, he knew we would also recommend him to others, so it was a mutually beneficial arrangement. The next day he would show us the hospital where, if successful, our baby would be delivered. He would also show us some apartments we could choose to stay in next time around, if there was a next time of course. Once arrangements for the next day were finalised Puneet left and we went on into the early hours very contentedly sipping several more Kingfishers.

19

INVESTIGATING MUMBAI

Breakfast was served daily outside in the small garden to the back of the hotel. The same waiters that had served us Kingfishers the night before now served us an Indian breakfast consisting of a copious amount of fruit, boiled eggs, omelettes cooked to order, breads, spicy sauces, salads, potatoes, juices, tea and coffee. Indian tea may well be renowned the world over but trying to get the coffee to suit our western taste was a futile exercise, and finally the waiter decided the easiest thing was to bring the coffee, a jug of boiling water, a jug of hot milk and the cups and let us off to make our own. Without ever having to ask again, the waiter carried out this ritual for us every morning. We sat outside every morning amongst the lush greenery and exotic plants and flowers. Birds as large as seagulls hovered over us ready to land in the middle of our table if we dared to leave our plate unattended. We were careful not to eat any salad or food that may have been washed in water. We only ate fruit that could be peeled and drank bottled water rather than the water provided in large jugs. We had been warned to check that the seal on water bottles was unbroken before buying, as many shops refilled water bottles with tap or rainwater to resell to the unsuspecting tourists. Over time we spotted this going on in many places and made sure we were extra vigilant.

Puneet arrived after breakfast and off we went for the day. Our first stop was going to be the hospital. We travelled across the city through filthy rubbish-strewn streets where people lay in rags on the ground. Animals and people were scavenging and fighting over one scrap of priceless food. We were fiercely reminded that we were in a city of contrasts as we approached an area known as Powai. It skirted around the beautiful lake and was extensively surrounded by perfectly manicured open spaces. Huge gates and high walls separated the lowly from immaculately maintained gardens with driveways leading to exclusive houses and top-class hotels. Dr L H Hiranandani Hospital was a private hospital located in this exclusive and upmarket district, an affluent area with security at every entrance to every public building including the hospital. Every person and every bag was subject to rigorous searching when either entering or leaving the buildings. It was reassuring because it wasn't that long ago that Mumbai was the target of terrorist bombings. 2010 was the last attack and ever since, high-level security was in place at entrances to all public places including shopping centres, offices, supermarkets, hotels and hospitals. Puneet checked with security to see if Edel could be allowed into the hospital to film, but she was refused. Only people who had an appointment or a specific reason for visiting the hospital were allowed entry. Puneet then explained to security the purpose of our visit. We were allowed in, but we had to give an undertaking that we would not attempt to take any photographs, and we would remain on the ground floor and not attempt to access any other part of the hospital.

The ground floor itself was vast, with a large sweeping staircase and several elevators to the upper floors. There were fourteen floors and what we gleaned from our brief and restricted visit was that it was extremely well maintained, clean and organised. Without seeing the rest of the building, we left reassured that it was a hospital with high standards. We felt that if Shobha became pregnant this was a hospital that we would be happy for her to be cared in.

After our hospital visit, Puneet brought us on to the Marriot and Ramada hotels a short distance away. Both hotels had apartments for rent within the complex and patrons could use all of the hotel facilities which ranged from a launderette to a gym, numerous restaurants, running track, pools, tennis courts and several walking trails through the extensive grounds. They were geared for the western tourist market. While certainly exclusive and safe, we had concerns in that firstly, they were more than double the price we were currently paying and secondly, we didn't know if we really wanted to live in a complex like this, sanitised of all Indian culture. Puneet was touting for business and placing great emphasis on the security aspect which of course is important, but not to the extent that we would end up seeing nothing of the real India we were both so eager to explore. The apartments themselves were quite small but well laid out and had everything one would need. Prices ranged from €150 per night. Do the maths and multiply that by six weeks – the minimum time we would be in Mumbai if we returned – and you end up with a bill of about €6,300 plus local taxes of 5 per cent, and that's before any additional costs for things like printing and Wi-Fi. Then we would need to live, to eat, travel, buy groceries, buy baby food, equipment and clothes and any other incidentals. It would be very costly to move into one of these hotels. We knew even then that they were a non-runner but at least we had knowledge of the higher-end options available to us ... should we win the Lotto. Most definitely we would be looking for cheaper options if returning.

20

EMBRYO TRANSFER

On Tuesday, 29 January, we got the call. They had harvested eight eggs and following fertilisation we had six viable pre-embryos as a result. They were all of good quality: four grade As and two Bs. Seán laughed on hearing this saying, 'four As and two Bs, sure I didn't get that in the Leaving Cert'. He still goes on about it to everyone and anyone. The transfer was scheduled for 10 a.m. the following morning. In the meantime, we had to decide what grade combination and how many pre-embryos we wanted to transfer to Shobha. When we met previously with Dr Kadam one of the questions we put to her was about the maximum number of pre-embryos that could be transferred to optimise chances of success. She had explained that the maximum the clinic would allow us to transfer was three, but if we were successful in a triple pregnancy the clinic would not allow the pregnancy to term because it would be too great a risk for both Shobha and the babies. In that case they would carry out what they called a 'reduction'. In other words, they would abort a foetus and reduce a triple pregnancy to a twin pregnancy.

Seán and I talked and talked about this dilemma. We felt that to transfer one embryo was not sufficient to give us a realistic chance of success. We were at a stage where we really needed to maximise our chances. We'd had five unsuccessful attempts at IVF, when each time we had transferred two pre-embryos. If we were to go with two pre-embryos again and if we were again unsuccessful, that would be the end for us. Our last chance and our last option would be gone. But how would we be able to deal with and accept a decision to reduce or abort one of our babies if it were a triple pregnancy? This was the policy of the clinic, but it presented a huge, profoundly emotional dilemma for us. Do we transfer three pre-embryos in the full knowledge that we could end up unsuccessful with no baby, or on the other end of the scale successful with a triple pregnancy and then the awful decision that such a pregnancy would demand? Whether one wants to call it a reduction or an abortion or any other clinical term, it doesn't matter, the end result is the same. The question is could we live with that?

We knew if a decision had to be made it would not be ours to make, but it would be something we would have to live with for the rest of our lives. We no longer had time on our side. We needed the best chance of success. On that basis we made the decision to transfer three pre-embryos. We really hoped for success with either a single or twin pregnancy so that we would never have to contemplate the clinic's decision.

It was the morning of 30 January. On our way to the clinic, we sat silently in the rickshaw contemplating what was ahead of us, what we had started and now had to finish. Both of us were trying to mask the inner anxiety and trying to be there for each other. This was it, this was the day, and after today there would be no turning back. Were we able to do this, a baby and everything that comes with that? As we slowly and deliberately climbed the stairs to the clinic, another group of women were sitting on the steps waiting for what they hoped would be their chance at a better life. We huddled together again in the small waiting area, holding hands, trying to pass strength through touch. Dr Kadam made her entrance, elegantly sweeping past us, dressed beautifully in her Indian sari accessorised with discreet pieces of jewellery. A palpable aura of importance enveloped her as she moved gracefully towards her office. The camera crew was set up and ready. It was one of those moments when we wished we hadn't allowed the TV crew to take over our lives.

She confirmed matter-of-factly that we had four grade A and two grade B pre-embryos. She also confirmed that we should transfer three pre-embryos for the best chance of success; two grade A and one grade B being the best combination. We already knew that three was the best number and her affirmation of that was all we really wanted. We didn't need any more discussion or persuasion. We'd had so much bad luck in the past we had no choice now but to go with the number and combination that gave us the best possible chance of success. We asked more questions concerning Shobha. How was she feeling that morning? Would her husband and children be able to visit her? Would she be able to leave the surrogate house at any stage? Shobha was in good spirits and happy to proceed, and of course her husband and children could visit her; arrangements were already made for visits every weekend. We looked through the pictures of the surrogate house on her computer, flicking between different rooms, all of which seemed bare and quite basic. But we knew that for Shobha this was better accommodation than she was used to. For the majority of surrogate mothers, the basic surrogate house was comparable to a five-star hotel. Indeed for more than 70 per cent of the population, it was a palace in comparison to what they were used to. For some to even have a roof over their heads was a luxury.

This residence, along with the provision of nutritious food, plenty of rest and medical care, also had a knock-on effect in that there would be more food to go around at home for the rest of the family. The surrogate mothers are often taught new skills such as sewing or embroidery while in the house, to better equip them to earn a living after they return home. We asked about Shobha's care while she would be in the surrogate house. It was explained that she would receive full medical care, monthly checks-ups and scans and whatever additional care or medications were needed. She would be visited daily by a doctor from the clinic as a matter of routine, and more frequently if she was unwell. She would be taken by taxi to and from the clinic for her check-ups and scans. We would know in advance when the scans and appointments at the clinic were scheduled so that we could arrange to Skype Shobha at the clinic. Some surrogate mothers wished to go home for festivals and special family occasions, but this was only allowed if permission was sought and given by the intending parents. Generally visits home were not encouraged. This was to ensure that the surrogate mother did not drink alcohol, take drugs, non-prescribed medications or even have unprotected sex which might place both herself and the baby at risk.

We were beckoned down the corridor by a uniformed staff member who pointed to some disposable gowns, masks, shoe covers and hats, indicating for us to put them on. Not quite sure why we were gowning up or where we were going, we still followed her instructions and allowed her to lead us on into the theatre. Shobha was lying on the trolley, gowned and covered up with a sheet. She was smiling but also looked nervous as she glanced at each of us in turn. I smiled at her in what I hoped was a reassuring way, though I felt not a bit reassured myself; all the emotions and anxieties were doing battle in my heart. Careful not to touch any equipment, we were led into a small annex where suddenly projected onto a screen for us to see, were our pre-embryos. It was a defining moment in time for us as we both stared at the screen unable to move, transfixed. They were our babies, our future.

And in the blink of an eye, as surreal as that moment was, it was gone. It was time for the transfer. Stepping outside, I couldn't speak because I knew if I did, I'd only start crying. It was overwhelming. Did these people really understand? Did Shobha really understand what they gave to people like us, the hope and chance of a family together? I could see Seán also finding it difficult to maintain his composure. Meanwhile, the camera was a witness to our struggle capturing our most vulnerable moments.

More composed, we waited until the nurse came to tell us that the transfer had been completed and there had been no problems. She handed us a summary sheet of the IVF Cycle outlining the details of the transfer. We were given 14 February, St Valentine's Day, as the next contact date. This was the date we would get confirmation as to whether the transfer had been successful and if we were going to have a baby or not. After about an hour of resting in the clinic, Shobha would be moved to the surrogate house, but if we wanted we could see her one final time before she was moved. I took Shobha's two hands in mine and gave them a gentle squeeze. We said nothing for no words were adequate.

The remainder of our time was spent doing everything that ordinary tourists do, visiting the sights of Mumbai. The Taj Mahal Palace hotel was opulence at its most magnificent. The Gateway of India, Elephant Island and the Hare Krishna Centre were all on our list of places to visit, as well as many of the bazaars and markets. We mingled with all the other tourists buying souvenirs as reminders of our trip as well as gifts for those at home. Near the Gateway of India, while wandering through the streets, Seán met a tailor plying his trade on the street. He went for it, and in minutes was being measured for a bespoke suit. The tailor told us to return in three hours. When we did, he presented Seán with a perfectly tailored Indian suit for fifty quid! We also got caught out by the young Indian girls 'giving away' small garlands of flowers, but no sooner was the garland placed around our necks and we were harassed until we handed over some money. You couldn't but admire their tenacity, but it's worth remembering there are no free lunches in India.

At night, we tried Indian fare in the many different restaurants washed down by cool bottles of Kingfisher beer. We whiled away the hours with Denise and Edel, chatting about how our day had gone. As the week drew to a close, we started to prepare for our return to Ireland. We had a long stopover on this leg of the journey, landing just after midnight in Dubai with our connecting flight not due to depart Dubai until after 7 a.m. We knew if we were making this journey any time again, we would have to sort out better flights with a lot less stopover time.

21

THERE WILL ALWAYS BE THREE

We were back home before people even realised we were gone and spent a long two weeks waiting for the results, every day dragging at a snail's pace, every day a mix of anxiety and excitement. It was difficult to talk about it because it was all just supposition at that stage, nothing was real. St Valentine's Day finally arrived. We knew the results had been emailed to us early that morning, but because Edel and Denise wanted to film us getting the results from Dr Kadam, we exercised extreme willpower and didn't go near the laptop. And like Murphy's Law, when we tried to connect on Skype we couldn't. Of all days! We had to abandon Skype and resort to phoning Dr Kadam. The phone had no loudspeaker function, so while talking to Dr Kadam I would have to try to relay the information as best I could to Seán. I punched in the numbers, this was it and this was the moment.

It was ringing. I heard a slight click as the receiver was picked up and the word, 'congratulations' sounded over the line. Oh my God, it had happened! Shobha was pregnant! I didn't have to say anything. Seán could read my expression. She must have thought me crazy as I just kept repeating what she had said, but I was trying to let Seán know what was happening. I asked if she knew if it was a single pregnancy or more. Before I had even finished the question, she replied, 'almost definitely multiple'. Multiple! Oh my God!

The conversation was over as quickly as it had started. We didn't ask anything else. We could email later but for now I just wanted to hug my man. Edel stopped filming and we all hugged each other. I knew both Denise and Edel were hoping for the documentary's sake that it would be good news, but I also knew that they were very happy for us. Donal's language was colourful to say the least, betraying his sheer delight for us. When we broke the news to him that it was possibly twins, he nearly swallowed his teeth.

We checked the email sent to us earlier that day. There it was, confirmed in black and white. It also detailed the next phase of the process for us. For the next four weeks there would be weekly blood tests and scans until there was definitive confirmation of whether it was a single, twin or triplet pregnancy. Going forward, we would then receive a full report and the scan images after every check-up. As the pregnancy progressed, Shobha would attend the clinic for monthly check-ups including blood tests and scans. In general, all the checks and scans carried out would be similar to what would be carried out during a pregnancy here in Ireland. If we didn't understand anything we were told to ask questions. In the meantime, if we had any queries we could email the clinic. Shobha was now back in the surrogate house where she would remain for the duration of the pregnancy. We were going to have a baby together. Life would never be normal again.

It's hard to write and I do so with a heavy heart. We were over the moon and took every opportunity to talk about our impending new family. A single pregnancy would be fantastic, but a twin pregnancy would be such a bonus. We never contemplated for a second that maybe it would be a triple pregnancy. I mean, surely after all our trying and failed efforts we couldn't be that fortunate and unfortunate at the same time.

The blood test results the following week showed the levels had increased to 8723 mIU/ml, confirming again that there was more than one baby, but still not indicating if it was twins or triplets. We would know for definite the following week. Again, Edel and Denise would be returning to Miltown to film us getting this news. This time we were able to get a connection to Skype. Dr Kadam immediately told us that the most recent scan showed three sacs. It was triplets. We were gobsmacked. What now? She informed us that they would wait for a few more weeks before making any decision; apparently sometimes there can be a spontaneous loss where triplets are expected. If this did not happen, however, they would have to carry out the reduction. I find it hard to even say the word 'abortion' but no matter what term or word is used to describe what may have to be done, either way it was extremely difficult for us to accept. We tried for so long to get pregnant, and now, ironically, we were being told we might have to terminate one foetus; it was so unfair. It was terrible to be hoping for a spontaneous abortion, but we did. We didn't want to face the consequences. We hoped and hoped, but each week the report came back telling us that 'all three foetuses were doing well'. Time for the reduction was drawing closer and while we are not religious people, I found myself pleading with my dead father and sister. I wanted Shobha to have a spontaneous termination. I'm sure Seán was doing the exact same, pleading with his mother and father. We got word that the 'foetal reduction' was scheduled for the next day, 6 April 2013. Even as I write this now, I try very hard not to let it in, but I feel the same pain and overwhelming sense of loss and sadness as I did on that day, and the tears come again, for the loss of our second child.

We weren't sure about the documentary presenting this particular piece to the nation. We had known the consequences if it was triplets, and we knew what we would be facing. We knew the decision would evoke much moral discussion in Catholic Ireland. Rightly or wrongly, people would judge us and criticise us. We would generate disapproval, anger and religious-based dissent, but above all else we were exposing ourselves to more hurt and pain. Did we really need to expose our vulnerability by airing this most personal hurt on national television? Edel and Denise felt it was a very important piece to include, but they also knew that any controversial issue would increase the viewership. Equally, this was not about Edel and Denise, this was about us and the loss of our baby, and it was our decision whether to include it or not.

We had agonising discussions, but ultimately came to the realisation that in agreeing to make the documentary we had a responsibility to be honest. We had to be honest, particularly for those people who might consider going this road. It was our decision to go public in the first place so that other people could see surrogacy as a very real option, but in doing so we also had a responsibility to present the full story, warts and all. We needed to give an honest account for the very same reason we agreed to make the documentary – so that couples could make informed decisions. It would have been very easy for us not to include this piece, but we are honest people and we had to allow its inclusion. On reflection maybe that was a mistake, but only in so far as it serves as a constant reminder. Do we need that reminder? No, we don't. For us, there will always be three.

22

PARENTAL LEAVE & LEGAL ISSUES

We could see our babies developing and growing each month, but in a kind of surreal way. I wasn't pregnant. I wasn't going through the experience of pregnancy, and we weren't having the usual check-ups associated with pregnancy. Instead we were relying on reports and scan results from another place and time. We worried constantly that all would be OK. Then we worried if we would bond and what if we didn't. We worried how we would manage with two babies. Would we have the energy for all this at our age? We had so many worries that at times we just frightened the shit out of ourselves.

Around this time in April 2013, I decided to inform my employer about the pregnancy and apply for leave. I had already told some close work colleagues, so this was logically the next step. It was also a scary move as there was no process, policy or procedure within my organisation to deal with any application for paid leave other than the usual maternity or adoptive leave. I knew well that as there was no legislation in Ireland governing surrogacy, there was no obligation on my employer to grant me paid leave. This was the uncertainty and inequity that we faced. It concerned me greatly at the time, as I knew I would be relying on the organisation's sense of fairness, equity and discretion in considering my application. I was deeply worried. If I didn't get leave, how was I going to go to India for anything up to eight weeks? How was I going to be able to spend time with my babies during the most important first year of their lives? The night before my meeting with my manager, I tossed and turned trying to figure out if he would support my application for leave or not, and what could I do if he didn't. If refused I would have to refer my case to the Equality Authority, but that wouldn't resolve the immediacy of needing leave, and I certainly couldn't afford to take unpaid leave, which of course might very well not be granted either.

I started by telling him about my changing family circumstances, how we had come to be where we were at, how we were expecting twins, and finally I made my request for leave. I was clear with him that there was no legislation on surrogacy in Ireland and as a result, there was no obligation on the organisation to grant me leave of any kind. But I explained that I was appealing to the organisation's sense of fairness and equity in this respect. I needn't have feared, as he was openly supportive. 'One is a parent by whatever means,' he said. I will never forget that response. I was over the first hurdle, but I knew I was by no means across the finish line, as other senior managers would also be signing off on my application. But no matter, I still left that meeting optimistic and on cloud nine. My manager, a senior manager in the organisation, was supporting me, and there may just be the possibility that I would be granted the leave.

It was also April when we went to see a solicitor who appeared to be the guru on surrogacy in this country. We were aware we would have legal issues to contend with on return to Ireland, and she confirmed a lot of what we already knew, giving us detailed information in an open and brutally honest way. The contract we signed was a legally binding agreement in India but not in Ireland, because there was no legislation. So, in effect, it wasn't worth the paper it was written on. We would not be recognised as parents and our babies would not be recognised as Irish citizens; they would be considered stateless. We would not automatically get passports for them or even visas to exit India. Instead, we would have to apply to the Irish passport office via the Irish embassy in India for emergency travel documents so that we could then seek exit visas to bring our babies home.

Once home, Seán, being the person with the genetic relationship to our children, would have to apply to the Circuit Court for a declaration of parentage and guardianship under the Children's Act 1977, and he would also have to seek leave to apply for passports for our children. For this application, we needed copies of all the legal documentation from India to be exhibited to the courts, and the Attorney General would have to be put on notice. She told us our case could be heard in Co Clare, our place of residence, or we could go to Dublin if we wanted. Once Seán was appointed guardian and legal custodian he would then need to update his will to name me as guardian intestate in the event of his death. Because of our government's failure to put legislation in place, the only way I would ever legally have custody or guardianship of our children was if Seán died.

She went on to explain that in the eyes of the state I would be non-existent because in our constitution the woman who gives birth is the legal mother. Therefore, in the eyes of the Irish state, the surrogate mother would be considered the mother of my children. I had thought naively that I too could apply to the courts to be recognised as their mother, given that both our names would be on the birth certificates. But no, she confirmed that despite the fact that I will look after our babies, care for them, love them and raise them, in Irish law I will not exist. I feel I shouldn't really care about that if I am doing everything a mother should be doing for her children, but of course I do, and of course I should. I passionately care that my children recognise me as their mother, and I know that they will. I know it will be a natural, loving and organic process and one that the Irish state cannot influence or prevent, but I also want to simply be recognised legally as their mother.

There was a schedule of documents we needed to bring back from India in order to issue proceedings in the Irish courts. These included:

- Birth certificates of the babies.
- Original surrogacy contract.
- DNA test results carried out by a reputable agency.
- Consent by the surrogate mother and if married, her husband to carry out DNA tests.
- Affidavit of doctor collecting DNA samples.
- Affidavit of marital status of surrogate and if married, affidavit of husband.
- If translations required, affidavit/Declaration of Advocate confirming that the translated documents have been explained to the surrogate and her husband if married.
- Affidavit regarding issuing of travel documents for both surrogate and husband if married.
- Affidavits regarding Sole Custody/Guardianship from both surrogate and husband if married.
- Proper permanent address for service on the surrogate mother and if married, her husband.

The costs involved in issuing court proceedings in Ireland would be in the region of €7,000 to €10,000. Again we were gobsmacked. We hadn't realised the cost would be so much. She went on to explain that immediately upon our return to Ireland we must initiate these legal proceedings; that was clearly stated in the Irish Guidelines. We didn't know where we would get the money to do so, but we would find it somewhere. We needed to take one step at a time. We left the meeting more than a little subdued, our buoyant upbeat mood having taken a bit of a hammering.

There had to be countless Irish families out there in the same situation, families that have been created through surrogacy. Many we realise may not have gone into court to ratify their situation, instead preferring to remain under the radar rather than risking the wrath of the Irish legal system. These parents and children are the casualties of our government's indifference. This has been allowed to happen because the Irish state, instead of dealing with surrogacy, historically ignore and procrastinate on controversial issues like this. They don't deal with them. Instead, they prefer to kick the can down the road or sweep them under the carpet. I know in my heart it will take forever to introduce legislation, and that's something I can barely contend with.

23

A VALUABLE ENCOUNTER

We managed to get the name and contact details of the Irish person who attended the Corion Clinic a couple of months before us. That person was now at home in Ireland with their baby and was currently going through the courts to ratify the situation. We made contact, hoping for a meeting as this was the first person we knew of that had been down this road. There was no hesitation in meeting with us and giving us whatever information and help we needed. For us it was invaluable just to be able to meet and talk to someone who had been through the process.

We got loads of information in terms of the logistics and everyday practicalities. Drawing a map for us, we were shown the approximate locations of the various offices we would need to visit in Mumbai: the Irish consulate, the clinic, the solicitor's office and the FRRO. Essential information and advice was given to us: the location of supermarkets close to the hospital; hiring a night nurse and the cost; the importance of recording minute details such as names, dates, times and signatures of the nannies or nurses hired to care for the babies. At a minimum, we were told we would need to make one trip to the Clinical Diagnostic Centre for the DNA test, one trip to the solicitor, two trips to the Irish consulate and one trip to the FRRO. We were advised about day-to-day living in India: what to watch out for and what to be careful with.

We didn't run with some of the information or advice given to us, such as bringing our own baby formula. I had done some research on this and knew that while India didn't have any of the formulas we have here in Ireland, they have a perfectly acceptable range available. In addition, despite needing an additional suitcase or two, it would be difficult to calculate the amount needed. Also, what if the formula didn't suit them? We'd end up being able to sell the stuff ourselves, so we had already decided at that stage to go with the formula available in India. I had checked the ingredients of the Indian formulas online and chose one that I felt would be close to one of the brands available in Ireland, so that when we returned home the transition wouldn't be too upsetting.

Worryingly, we were told how this person's baby had arrived earlier than planned, resulting in a panic to reorganise everything such as additional leave from work and flights. While eventualities such as this can happen, we knew we needed to ensure we got accurate dates to minimise the risk of missing the birth.

If we took anything away from this meeting it was the realisation of how important it is for anyone going through surrogacy to be able to meet or talk to others who have gone through the process, if only to get practical information and advice. We knew after the documentary went out we would make ourselves available to anyone considering surrogacy, to give what we had received – help, information and support.

24

TO VISA OR NOT TO VISA

Now implemented, the new Indian Visa Guidelines outlined in detail what was required of Irish people seeking to enter India. More specifically, they outlined what was required for people entering India for the purposes of a surrogacy arrangement. The document stated that all intending parents must now apply for a medical visa as opposed to a tourist visa, and it outlined the criteria to be eligible to apply for the medical visa.

We read and re-read the document and became increasingly worried, as we knew we couldn't comply with some of the criteria. Two criteria in particular concerned us:

1. 'The intending couple had to be married for at least two years.' We would be required to produce a marriage certificate as evidence that we had been married for at least two years.
2. 'That the child or children born to commissioning couples through surrogacy in India would be permitted to enter their country as their biological child/children.'

We, as the commissioning couple, would be required to produce evidence of this; at the very least, a letter from the Irish embassy in India or the Department of Foreign Affairs in Dublin reaffirming Ireland's position in relation to surrogacy in Ireland and specifically that Ireland recognised surrogacy.

One could only assume that these criteria were implemented because the Indian government had concerns about babies born in India through surrogacy to commissioning couples from countries that did not legally recognise surrogacy. The concern being that if the country in question did not recognise surrogacy in law, then the children may not be allowed into the country and the Indian authorities may be left to care for them.

The Irish authorities, in response, issued a briefing on these guidelines, which, amongst other things, stated:

> There are currently no circumstances in Ireland where a child born through surrogacy will be recognised here as the biological child of the commissioning couple ... The only way a child born through surrogacy in India can enter this country is if the commissioning male is Irish and an Irish Court Order has been obtained declaring him to be the parent of the child. This will permit the Irish authorities to issue a travel document or passport for the child.

What did this mean? While Seán would be the commissioning male, it appeared that he would have to go to court in Ireland in advance of being able to bring our babies home. It meant I would have to remain in India alone with our babies while Seán returned to apply to the courts for the order. It wasn't clear how long this would take or how long we would have to wait for a court hearing date. Could we be refused the court order and if so what then? If we did get a court order, it seemed Seán could then return to India to seek the travel certificates and exit visas. It was ambiguous, and it also seemed to be a complicated, convoluted and lengthy process, not to mention the costs involved. We had the concern that if we applied for the medical visas to the Indian embassy, we could be refused on the basis of not meeting the criteria. If this happened, we would not be able to travel to India at all; we would not be able to bring our babies home. What would happen to our babies in India? Would they end up in an orphanage? It was a bloody mess and we were right in the middle of it. Confused and afraid, we had nowhere to turn to for advice or information.

Our only port of call was the Irish embassy in New Delhi. I couldn't get through to them by phone, so on 24 June I emailed instead, outlining our intention to travel to India later in the year to bring home our twin babies born through surrogacy. I asked what documents were required of us and also about the DNA testing. What I was really hoping for was a solution to the medical-visa dilemma but instead we got a brief response which was even more confusing and ambiguous, if that was even possible. Rather than allay our fears, it raised even more concerns for us, as it stated that:

> In the absence of domestic surrogacy legislation it is not possible to provide a letter indicating that Ireland recognises surrogacy. Furthermore, it is not possible to indicate that the child will be permitted entry into Ireland 'as a biological child of the couple commissioning surrogate' since, as indicated on page two of the surrogacy guidelines, under Irish law the woman who gives birth to the child is the child's legal mother.

We were advised to read and adhere strictly to the Indian Visa Guidelines and the Irish Surrogacy Guidelines. There was no indication that we would get a medical visa if we applied, and there was no guidance, advice or support from our embassy in India. As a result, we made the decision to apply for a tourist visa for fear of being refused the medical visa. We knew at the time it was wrong, and we knew it would be inevitable that at some point we would be taken to task and penalised in some way for this decision, but we felt we were left with absolutely no choice.

The only comment the Irish embassy made to our query about the DNA testing was simply to state, 'DNA testing can only be carried out by the Ormond Quay Paternity Services (www.oqps.ie). You will need to contact them to arrange this in advance of the birth'.

Everything is great in hindsight, but we should have been forewarned by this response from our embassy in India regarding the level of support we would get from them when we returned to India later in the year.

25

DNA TESTING

The Irish Surrogacy Guidelines requires DNA testing to be done while in India to determine parentage. By confirming Seán as the biological father we would then be able to apply for the emergency travel certificates. Prior to contacting the Irish embassy in Delhi, and initially when we read this requirement, we weren't entirely sure how to go about arranging for a DNA test to be carried out in India, so we did the obvious and contacted the Corion Clinic. In response, they said they could arrange for the test to be carried out in a reputable clinic in Mumbai and have the samples transported to a DNA Diagnostic Centre in America for testing. However, we now knew that was a non-runner as per the response from the Irish embassy, and instead we made contact with the only Irish-approved clinic, the Ormond Quay Paternity Services (OQPS) in Dublin. We told them where we were at in the whole process and that we needed to arrange to have DNA testing done while in India. They talked us through each stage of the process:

1. We should contact their clinic again about four weeks before travelling to India to initiate the process.
2. We would be required to pay an initial deposit of €750.
3. Sampling kits would then be sent by OQPS to the clinic in India and preliminary arrangements made for testing.
4. Contact details of the clinic and doctor in India would be sent by email to us.

5. We should phone the clinic when our babies were born to arrange the test.

6. We should attend the clinic for testing with our babies.

7. A witness from the Irish embassy would be in attendance.

8. Seán's passport, his passport photos and our babies' passport photos would be required.

9. The embassy witness would confirm Seán and our babies' identification.

10. The doctor would take the samples.

11. Samples would then be transported back to OQPS in Dublin.

12. OQPS would send the samples on to the UK for testing.

13. Paternity testing would be carried out.

14. Results would be sent back to OQPS in Dublin from the UK.

15. Final payment should be made to the clinic.

16. Results would then be emailed to us.

17. Results would also be issued to the passport office, the Irish embassy and the Irish consulate.

18. We would make the application for emergency travel documents.

19. The Irish passport office would sanction emergency travel certificates.

20. Emergency travel documents would be issued.

They outlined a couple of turnaround time options available to us. There was a regular turnaround time for results of up to fourteen days or alternatively the testing could be fast-tracked in forty-eight hours for which we would pay an additional cost. It was explained that because the samples needed to be transported from India to Dublin and on to the UK, and in turn, the results had to be sent from the UK to Dublin and then on to us, all in all the process could still take anywhere from forty-eight hours to two weeks before we would have results. So what did they mean by fast track? Was there really only one clinic in Ireland equipped to provide this service or was there another reason for this monopoly?

The complete testing process cost us €1,600. One couple told us that in only one year following our return, costs for this test had increased to €2,575 – a 76 per cent increase. This is probably as a result of increasing numbers of Irish people going abroad for surrogacy, and maybe also because for whatever reason, there is no competition in providing this service.

26

TELLING

The documentary was progressing, and every few weeks or so Denise and Edel travelled down to Miltown to film where we were at. It was really time to start telling people, but this was something we had been putting off for a while. I, especially, was fast approaching my biggest fear: telling my sons, Diarmáid and Rián. I didn't know how they would react, and I was afraid that they would feel less wanted or loved; something that couldn't have been further from the truth. I was worried they would be angry or embarrassed that their mother was having more children ... at our age. I knew telling them would have to be faced sometime, but I kept putting off the inevitable. I also knew I couldn't settle and wouldn't be content until we had told them. We all needed time to get our heads around this, and they were no different, so it wouldn't have been fair to spring it on them at the last minute. It had to be done. Building up the courage, we decided how best to approach the subject with them, as it was now early July and it was getting too close for comfort. It was now or never. We called them to the kitchen saying we needed to talk.

The first thing Diarmáid asked was, 'What have we done?'

'Nothing,' we replied. 'It's what we've done.'

And then we just told them straight out. We were going to India to bring home twin babies. We didn't at that point say it was surrogacy because we didn't want to overload them. They needed time to absorb what we had just told them before we broached the subject of surrogacy. Diarmáid said he had an inkling something like that was going to happen while Rián was quieter in his response, but they both seemed happy for us. They didn't tell us we were an embarrassment nor did they scream at us for being irresponsible adults, instead they asked us some questions and we discussed things openly. The relief for us both, especially me, was immeasurable. We told the boys if they had any questions to come back and ask us. Our intention, in a week or so, when they had digested the news was to sit down again with them and explain about surrogacy. Now we could start to tell our close friends and family.

The following week Diarmáid and Rián did ask about the babies. They had lots of questions, often catching me completely unawares: did we meet the mother when we were in India in January and why was she giving up her babies? It was obvious they thought it was adoption, a natural conclusion for them to come to. So earlier than planned, and again with niggling worries about how they would take it, we sat down and told them about surrogacy: what it was and how it had worked for us. We explained it all to them and they surprised us again by accepting the whole concept of surrogacy so readily and in a completely non-judgemental manner. Sometimes as adults we are quick to criticise our young people unfairly for their lack of understanding, when really they can be far more open-minded and non-judgemental than the adult academic or well-educated population.

Telling our close friends provoked various reactions, from the obvious shock and horror, to being absolutely and completely dumbfounded. We suffered a few sympathetic looks implying we were lost causes, but in all cases our friends were genuinely happy for us but equally glad it wasn't them. We were also equally sure that when the shock dissipated, the opinion that we were mad would linger … and for a very long time we suspected. Edel wanted to film us telling some friends or family, to catch the moment and the reaction live. We arranged to visit Mairéad and David knowing full well the reaction would be magnificent and worth capturing. We told them there was a programme being made about Irish music and that the film crew wanted a chance to record a session in a home situation. Mairéad was completely nonplussed but agreed. Well, it was so worth it for her reaction alone. She surpassed all our expectations, cursing so much that it had to be edited out of the documentary in the end but what couldn't be edited out was their genuine elation and happiness for us; it was so sincere it was humbling.

Over the next few weeks we were busy telling all our close friends. Emer and Mike already knew. We visited Mary and Scruff and then Breda and Tony who provided us with one of our funniest reactions. Tony, when initially told, sat silently lost in thought and surprisingly said very little indeed. The next day he phoned and told us that he had woken up at about 4 a.m. in a lather of sweat only just realising what we had said. He had been in shock until then.

It started to become easier. Seán told Noel, his close friend and partner at work, and then he told the lads he played with in the band one evening, just as they prepared to play a gig. Máire and Tom were told the same evening during a break in the music. Soon, all but my 82-year-old mother knew. She was well known for her quick, caustic tongue and was certainly not one to pull any punches when she had something to say. I had to tell her, but every time I thought of it, the dread would build up inside me and I would put it off for another time.

Then Christine, my sister, announced she was arriving. You'd swear it was designed and that she knew we had something to tell her. She arrived from Australia for a visit one week or so ahead of her daughter Aisling and her husband, John. The easiest thing was to take the opportunity to tell her first and let her do the explaining then to John and Aisling. I still remember the shock on her face and her efforts to disguise it, while at the same time admitting to us that she could never go back to baby days again. At the same time, she expressed her admiration for us in going after what we wanted in life. Christine, never one to be shy of the camera, participated in the documentary wholeheartedly, like a duck to water.

It was time. I had to tell my mother, and Seán was coming along for the ride and to give me much needed support. As it turned out, telling her was insignificant, like telling her we were going away on holidays. There was no grand inquisition, no horrified look, no 'are ye mad' comments, just acceptance that we were doing what we wanted to do. She asked us in doing what we were doing were we hurting anyone, to which we said no. She then asked if we were happy, to which we replied yes. 'Well, isn't that what matters,' she said.

Seán had taken to letting people know we might not be around during September and October. As he put it, 'we have a couple of projects' to attend to. No one really asked what these projects were, as everyone and anyone who knows Seán knows he could be organising anything from a presidential Sinn Fein visit to a U2 rock concert in the Fairgreen. Maureen, a close friend, to this day always asks after 'the projects'.

As we edged closer to the expected date, we continued to get the monthly reports and scans knowing that very soon we would be getting them every two weeks. Things were progressing as normal and our babies were gaining weight and developing as they should. Shobha was also doing very well and not experiencing any problems. By mid-August we were told our babies were due around 26 September, but still there was no definite date given. Being Irish, and with a slightly superstitious nature, I had bought nothing yet in preparation for the arrival. I still knew we had to be practical and be somewhat organised and ready. I couldn't just wait until we were home to start looking for cribs and sterilisers and baby clothes, so I trawled Done Deal to see it I could get some bargains. I was lucky. I spotted someone selling two cots and two cribs. They were identical and looked immaculate, and better still she was living in Co Clare. So off I went to collect them, easily pretending they were for a friend. Then Mairéad, the fountain of knowledge on all things baby decided we were going to hit Mothercare for the remaining essentials. Confidently, she guided us through the aisles picking up this and that, giving her expert opinion on the various brands. At that surreal moment, suddenly everything became very real: we were going to have twins and here I was with so much to do, so much to get and too much to choose from. How could I know what I really needed? What could I put off until we returned and what was a luxury that we could do without? Things had changed so much since I was a much younger and much more confident mother.

The spare room had turned into a store room for all things baby. It was full of baby equipment: blankets, tiny hats, mittens and socks, bibs, muslin cloths, Babygros, towels, talcum powder ... was talcum powder still used I wondered. I had it anyway, just in case, and I still have it! Nappies, wipes and Sudocream were all ready for our return as well as soothers, thermometers and of course, Calpol. The room was like a fortress with the curtains closed and the door locked in case an unexpected visitor dropped by. It would have been too tricky trying to explain that one away. We were so careful to ensure that no one other than our close inner circle of friends and family knew what we were doing. This was all down to fear. A fear that if anyone else were to find out about our plans they might, inadvertently or otherwise, tell someone who might let it slip to the 'authorities', and we might be stopped from bringing our babies home. We couldn't take the chance that anyone outside that inner circle would find out before we got to India.

27

LOGISTICAL DECISIONS & IMPORTANT PREPARATION

Our solicitor in India, who was recommended by the clinic, replied very promptly to our email. She told us what documents we needed to bring with us, what she would be doing for us and her fees. We were to bring:

- Our original birth certificates.
- Proof of residency such as any title certificate or mortgage contracts.
- Utility bills in joint names.
- Proof of citizenship such as passports.
- Visas.
- Joint bank account details.
- Divorce/separation agreements.
- Additional photo ID such as driving licences.
- The signed original surrogacy contract.

The documents had to be attested, and we were to bring several copies of each. She outlined her fee, which reassuringly was a set fee and would not change irrespective of any difficulties encountered. We could pay when we met in India, which again was reassuring not to have to send money in advance to someone we didn't know or had not yet met. She confirmed we would be in India for a minimum of six weeks. From her experience, it would take that long to get all the paperwork in place and obtain the emergency travel certificates and exit visas for our babies. We made final arrangements to meet with her in her office the first week we arrived in India.

From the get-go we had been talking about names. Once born and while still in hospital, we would need to register our babies and so we needed to have the names decided. Indian law does not allow the gender to be divulged in advance of the birth and while we loved the surprise element, it meant we had to be prepared for any combination: two boys, two girls or one of each. After lots of musing and eliminating we finally settled on two boys' and two girls' names, and if we did end up having one of each then we would just go with the first name in each set.

Meanwhile, we had been researching our accommodation options for our next stint in India. The three-star hotel we had stayed in previously was still pricey for what we were getting. The room was tiny and facilities were minimal. On the plus side, we already knew it was in a good location and the staff were nice and friendly. However, with two babies, the room would be too small and it would cost a lot more for a larger room. The lack of communal indoor and outdoor space remained a concern. Cabin fever would definitely be an issue. On the other hand, hotels and apartments with more facilities and bigger rooms were a lot more expensive, so we decided that while we were on our own initially, we would stay in the three-star hotel we knew, and when we had our babies with us we would then move to an apartment in Pune, a city three hours' drive south of Mumbai and recommended by the Australian couple as a very good but much cheaper option to Mumbai.

Pune is a young university city and not as built up or chaotic as Mumbai and supposedly it had plenty shops, restaurants and lots of accommodation to choose from. The couple also recommended Rajesh Dadhe, a man whom they knew and who rented out apartments. After checking with the clinic to ensure it was OK for us to go to Pune, they agreed there was no specific reason for us to stay in Mumbai after the birth. The clinic also confirmed that other people attending the clinic had gone to stay in Pune following the birth with no problems. We then contacted two couples who knew Rajesh. One couple had stayed in his apartment and another couple were currently using the accommodation. Full of praise, the UK couple described it as a spacious three-bedroomed apartment, basic but clean. They also said that Rajesh, the owner, lived upstairs which was helpful if there were any problems, and he had a wealth of contacts if anything was needed. They described Pune as a safe, clean, modern city where the climate was not as hot or oppressive as Mumbai. There were many hypermarkets, all well equipped with modern necessities. Many parks were easily accessible, the nearest only ten minutes away from the apartment. Everything sounded good, so our final check was with our solicitor in India to see if she needed us to stay in Mumbai for any specific reason after the birth; she didn't. Whatever we needed to get done, she assured us, could be done during the first week while in Mumbai. After that, communication could be via email with courier services being used if we needed to send or receive documents.

We decided to travel to Mumbai four or five days in advance of the birth and during that time we would travel to Pune. We would settle in to the apartment and buy what we needed, so that we would be all set up when we returned with our babies. We would then return to Mumbai the day before the birth. Rajesh offered us the same apartment that the other couples had used and told us the kitchen was equipped with a washing machine, fridge and cooker. It also had the essentials such as a microwave and kettle. We knew that these everyday kitchen items were not common in houses or apartments in India, so it was very important to specify well in advance what our requirements were and then of course to follow up and ensure they were in place before arriving. He assured us that everything we required would be provided, and we would also have security, a housekeeper and a cook as part of the deal. Free Wi-Fi and use of a fax and printer would also be provided and all for Rs. 3,170 (€45) a night. Later, he informed us that the longer we stayed, the cheaper the price became. If we stayed three weeks or more, it would cost Rs. 2,200 (€35) a night. He could arrange a nanny for €4 or a nurse for €8 for a full eight-hour shift. He could also arrange for a local car and driver at €17 per day. It was brilliant, too good to pass up and way cheaper than anything we could have got in Mumbai. We booked it immediately. Any of the well-known hotels we had seen with Puneet in Mumbai cost at least €100 per night, while the self-catering apartments cost up to €141 per night, excluding all of the extras that Rajesh was offering.

The next step was organising our flights. I tried to get the clinic to confirm the expected date of birth or at least as near as possible to the birth. While we wanted to be in India a few days in advance to get organised, we didn't want to be there for too long in advance, using up our precious leave. The expected date remained 26 September 2013, which was the end of week 37. Obviously we worried that Shobha might go into labour earlier than expected, and of course we had the typical questions. Would it be a natural birth or a caesarean section? Would Shobha be admitted to hospital earlier than usual? Would our babies remain in hospital for longer than normal? We had the very same worries that any parent expecting a baby might naturally experience; we were no different in that respect.

Pushing for more information, we emailed the clinic again, explaining to Dr Kadam that we were planning on arriving in India on 25 September. This was a white lie, as we really intended to arrive four or five days in advance, but I wanted them to realise that if the birth date was brought forward for any reason, we might not be in India for the birth. This time the clinic came back to us and said that because it was twins they believed it would be a caesarean section, but they would confirm this with the hospital. They also said that if it was a section they could, on our behalf, request 26 September to be confirmed as the birth date. We jumped at this. And some short time later, 26 September 2013 was confirmed as the date our children would enter the world.

We were flying with British Airways on 21 September 2013, with our return flight booked for six weeks later on 1 November. We decided this time to fly from Shannon to Heathrow with Aer Lingus and connect with British Airways from Heathrow direct to Mumbai. It was more expensive to take this route in comparison to flying with Emirates via Dubai, but as we would be returning with two small babies we needed to ensure the journey was as stress free and as easy as possible. We certainly didn't want to be landing in Dubai in the middle of the night again for a long stopover. The stopover in Heathrow would be four hours. This gave us enough time on the return leg to get from terminal five to terminal one, to change from summer to winter clothes, to feed and change the babies and to allow for any delays.

About this time I also contacted OQPS in Dublin again, the service responsible for the DNA testing. We paid the deposit to initiate the process, following which, they confirmed that they had sent the kits to Mumbai and gave me the contact details of the doctor in the Clinical Diagnostic Centre. We were to make contact with the doctor after the birth to arrange for the samples to be taken.

Then, just three weeks before we were due to fly, we got an email from Rajesh about our accommodation in Pune. The family currently in the apartment had to stay longer than expected, and unfortunately it was no longer available to us. He recommended another apartment owned by his friend, Abhijeet. He said this apartment would also have all the equipment we required, but we would not have the cook and housekeeper. It would have security and we could still organise for a car and driver or a nanny at the rates he had quoted if we wished. He said it was in a good area near to shops and supermarkets, so while we were disappointed, this apartment sounded quite similar and as it was more or less the same price we went ahead and booked it. We didn't have the luxury of time to go and start looking all over again.

The hospital where Shobha was due to give birth now required an advance payment of Rs. 75,000 (€1,000) as deposit for Shobha and our babies' birth, treatment and care. This was standard procedure and would be offset against our final bill, which we would be required to settle prior to being discharged with our babies. The final bill would increase if there were any complications, for example, if one or both of our babies' required neonatal care or any additional medications, or if Shobha needed any extra care. It was confirmed that our bill would be itemised on a daily basis for us, so we knew exactly what we were paying for.

Some unexpected and very worrying news arrived on 16 September, very shortly before we were due to fly out. Shobha had been admitted to hospital with threatened preterm labour. She had been transferred during the night to the hospital with abdominal pain, and they were monitoring her condition. We got such a shock. I suppose she had come so far with no problem whatsoever that we had relaxed and just never expected this. Thinking of Shobha and the babies the worry was intense. Despite reassurances that she was stable, we still couldn't help but be very concerned and wondered if we should arrange to fly out earlier. Emailing back and forth anxiously looking for more information and reassurance was not ideal, but Dr Kadam responded saying there was no need for us to travel early. Everything was fine for the moment, but we should be prepared to travel earlier just in case. They would keep us up to date daily as events progressed.

I started packing hastily, glad I had a list to consult to make sure we didn't forget anything. It was extensive and included all the usual suspects: mosquito repellent, mobile phones and chargers, adaptors, camera, laptop and iPad, a list of 'just in case' medications, pens and pads and an external hard-drive with every bit of communication and information regarding surrogacy saved on it. I ticked off each item until finally everything except the last-minute items were packed. We were ready.

I proceeded to print off several copies of all the documents we would need. The bank had been notified that we would be in India for up to six weeks to ensure our bank cards wouldn't be frozen while away. Diarmáid and Rián were catered for, and as well as filling the freezer with food, we gave them money to cover day-to-day costs. We gave the emergency fund to Emer and Marion in case the boys ran out, which of course they did! We couldn't be more ready. The now twice-a-day updates continued to state that Shobha 'remained stable'. Our babies seemed determined to hold on for us.

The day before we were due to fly was my mother's birthday, 82 years young. We tried to fit so much into that day: visiting her for her birthday, stocking up on last-minute supplies of grocery shopping and most importantly, spending time with Tomás, Diarmáid and Rián. We had a birthday cake for my mother, and as we had the craic she gave us a dire warning telling us not to return without a girl, so no pressure! That night we went to a local pub to meet up with our close friends for a discreet farewell, and we had our last bit of savage craic in Ireland for a while.

28

RETURNING TO INDIA

Next morning and up at cock-shout, Seán rounded up the cattle and got them inside handy enough except for the one red-white head and her calf, who took off over the land and out of sight the minute she spotted Seán. Try as he might he couldn't locate them and eventually gave up the ghost. Breakfast was a busy affair, as our close friends all landed to wish us well on the journey. Donal then arrived and he and Seán went off to sort out some final jobs on the farm; Donal would be in charge until our return. Thankfully on the way back home they found the red-white head and her calf, which was a relief. All cattle were now safely inside and although a bit earlier than other years, they would remain there for the winter. Saying goodbye to Tomás was particularly difficult for Seán and even more so because this would be the longest period of time they would ever have been apart. I knew he worried greatly about Tomás.

With the car loaded to the gills, we drove slowly through town for a last look around and then out the other end for the most adventurous and terrifying journey of our lives. When we arrived at Shannon we were told we couldn't check our baggage all the way through to Mumbai because we were booked onto two separate airlines. More worryingly for us, it seemed it would be the same for our return journey. We wondered how in the name of God we would manage the journey home with two babies and all the paraphernalia that comes with them. But we didn't have the time to think about that then. We had too much else to focus on, and it was just about time for a couple of parting glasses in the bar.

We had three hours before our connecting flight departed from Heathrow, and almost immediately we saw the enormity of the problem facing us on the return journey. We would have to get from terminal five to terminal one on the underground train with luggage, babies, buggy and God knows what else. Pushing the problem to the back of our minds for another day, we checked in and went off in pursuit of Denise and Edel and a bit to eat before departure. The flight itself was easy in comparison to our first trip via Dubai. Although Emirates was more comfortable and luxurious than British Airways, from a logistics perspective we had no long stopover, and we knew we had made the right decision.

Following a somewhat rough approach, we landed in Mumbai around 11.30 a.m. on Sunday, 22 September. Already you could see the wavering shimmer of heat on the concrete. It was blistering hot. Before emerging from the airport, we stopped at the same currency exchange booth as last time to change currency. We knew from our first trip that rupees could not be bought in advance in Ireland. We also knew that the airport rates were not only competitive, but they would buy back any rupees, commission free, before departure. The more currency you bought the better the rate; so on that basis we changed €2,000. We guessed we would be changing a lot more by the time we were ready for home.

Getting through immigration was as chaotic as ever. As we walked away from the dour-looking, bespectacled man at the desk and headed towards the exit, we realised we were back in the mayhem and madness of it all. Chaos embraced us, and it seemed that time had just stood still and nothing had changed. Weaving our trolleys this way and that, through the masses of travellers, we edged our way slowly towards the exit where we hoped to locate our taxi. Our driver, sent by Rajesh, was there holding a piece of cardboard with my name written on it.

Outside, the dust rose in the dry heat as the cars and rickshaws raced along the streets narrowly missing each other. Beggars took their lives in their hands as they moved amongst the traffic. With thin wrinkled hands, palms upwards, they sought coppers in vain. Nothing had changed. We were soon on our way to Pune to settle into the apartment and buy what we needed before returning to Mumbai for the birth. Pune is a three and a half hour drive southwards on the Mumbai highway, which is considered to be a very dangerous and fast stretch of road renowned for fatal, daily accidents. As we drove, we spotted bits of lorries and cars strewn along the side of the road. It was a frightening reminder of the dangers of driving in and around Mumbai. We were soon distracted from this as we feasted on the sights and scenery around us. The land was surprisingly beautiful with rich, green and lush pastures not unlike our own countryside. Cattle, goats and some sheep dotted the landscape, and they seemed to be the main benefactors of this farmland. There was some tillage and one could imagine that anything would grow in these unexpectedly lush valleys. It was still the rainy season and the combination of moisture and heat had the place bursting with growth and colour. We reached the outskirts of Pune at about 15.45 p.m. and made our way to what was to be our new home for the next six weeks.

29

PROBLEM-SOLVING
IN PUNE

Pune, pronounced 'Poona', is a modern business and academic city with a thriving university and IT hub. There is an abundance of apartment blocks, shopping centres, restaurants, bars and nightclubs, all doing a strong trade every night of the week. It's a city that looks like any other city the world over, but beneath the glossy exterior there is a level of deprivation and poverty lurking as was evident in Mumbai.

In contrast to its modern IT hub, Pune is also home to the renowned Soho International Meditation Resort attracting visitors from all over the globe with prices reflecting its international popularity. Pune has its own airport from which domestic flights arrive and take off frequently throughout the day. It is also home to the upscale northern suburb of Oregano Park, where one can while away the time in one of the many top-class hotels and shopping malls or maybe just take time out for a stroll.

Shopping centres or malls as they are called in India are plentiful and vast in both Mumbai and Pune; American influence is very evident. Malls generally have three to five floors with hundreds of shops selling both western and Indian goods. Like Mumbai, there is tight security everywhere, at entrances and exits to every hotel, shop and restaurant. No one is exempt from being searched. All bags are either stored by security until one is exiting or they are scanned and searched before people are allowed to enter with them. All cars entering hotels or other public buildings are subjected to security checks. The undercarriage of the vehicle is scanned using a mirrored telescopic device, and the boot of the car is also scrutinised.

Pune is a reminder of Ireland during the Celtic Tiger era when there was an abundance of cranes across our landscape. In Pune there are hundreds of them reaching to the sky as evidence of the vast amount of construction work going on in the city. Hotels, apartment blocks and more shopping centres go up every day. Pune is a city under serious development.

As we drove in the direction of our apartment, we noted that the area of the city we were in was relatively new and still very obviously under construction. We stopped outside a block of apartments and emerged from the car amidst rising dust from the unfinished road. Abhijeet, the apartment owner, along with his pal Rajesh greeted us. There were two or three more young men sitting around the entrance examining us intently. We made our introductions and then Rajesh introduced the staring men to us. They would be looking after us during our stay. They would organise anything we needed from shopping to takeaway meals. Directly across from our apartment block was yet another block still under construction. It was obvious our apartment was only recently finished, probably for our arrival. We knew immediately we would not be able to go for walks outside with the babies because the road itself was still unfinished and certainly not fit for a car let alone a buggy. Other concerns emerged too, for example, the apartment appeared to be very isolated. We hadn't seen any restaurants or shops in the immediate vicinity with the exception of one lone pharmacy that we had spotted as we turned into the road leading up to our apartment. There were no cars parked in the area, and we couldn't see any comings or goings which would indicate people actually working or living in the area. It seemed to us that there were very few other occupied apartments around us.

Abhijeet and Rajesh, watching us look around and sensing our concern, were very keen to reassure us about the area and particularly the isolation. They told us we would not need to leave the apartment as the staring men would get us whatever we needed: our meals, groceries, everything. That comment only worried us more, but we went on into the apartment to have a look, hoping that where we were going to live would be a place we would be delighted not to have to leave. Disappointingly, while it was very new and clean, it was also a shoebox with one bedroom containing only a double bed and bedside locker. There wasn't even space for either a wardrobe or dressing table. In fact, we weren't even sure there would be space for a crib in the bedroom let alone a cot. Our suitcases would have to be stored here, which I feared would cause mobility problems. The bathroom was even smaller, if that were possible, and certainly far too small for a baby bath to fit in. The sitting room had a coffee table, a sofa, one armchair and a TV fixed on the wall, with no space for anything else. An annex off the sitting room housed a brand new washing machine, obviously bought for our impending arrival. The kitchen boasted a fridge, sink, kettle, two cups, two plates, two forks and two spoons. That was it! No cooking facilities at all! There was no cooker or microwave, no kitchen table or chairs and again little or no space for anything else.

The view from the front window was the half-finished apartment block across the street. Our concern then shifted from the lack of space and equipment to the potential disruption that the noise emanating from the building works might cause. Meanwhile, to the rear of the apartment, the only window was in the annex and overlooked waste ground. Apparently this whole area was farmland up to a couple of years previous when the city began to develop. Apartment building was the focus of the construction industry in an endeavour to provide accommodation for the multinational IT corporations and their employees, but consequently there was little or no infrastructure in place.

I sat on the bed and my heart sank even more for the mattress was as hard as a rock. Our hearts in our boots, Seán and I glanced at each other. We both knew that this was not going to work for us, but we said nothing. We had very little time and we couldn't panic, not just yet. We needed to talk things through and decide.

Rajesh knew by us that we were worried. He tried to reassure us again that when the apartment in his block became available we could move there, but when we pressed him for a date he couldn't be definitive. The current tenant still did not know how long more she would need to stay in India. Rajesh hurriedly left us to settle in saying he would return in the morning to arrange for us to go to the shops to buy the baby equipment we needed. Once they left we just looked at each other. We didn't need to say anything; we both knew this wouldn't work for us. We needed this now like a hole in the head. In a few days our twins would be born. We had to be absolutely ready for them. We couldn't rely on the other apartment becoming available to us, but we also didn't know if we had the time to locate somewhere more suitable in a city we didn't know. But we had no choice, we had to try.

Powering up the laptop, we immediately set about searching for another place to live. The baby shopping arranged for the next day would have to go on the long finger. At the same time, we were hoping that Shobha would hold on and not deliver our babies early. Everything had been going so well that it was just too good to be true. Denise and Edel were staying at a local hotel, the Orchid, so with our tail between our legs we headed off to meet up with them for dinner and to break the news. Edel and Denise had planned to film us shopping the next day, but that was now scuppered. Instead, they would be rallying in behind us to help us in our quest.

By early morning, on my birthday, we had identified some properties that we wanted to view. By the time Denise and Edel arrived at 10 a.m. we had the address of four apartments we were going to visit. However, trying to phone and arrange viewings was another story due to the language barrier, but out of the four we managed to tie down three viewings. It would take all day because the traffic in Pune was very similar to that of Mumbai, incessant and congested.

We hired a taxi for the day and headed to the first viewing, which was a disaster. Located in a busy but very run down area of the city, the apartment itself was dirty with obvious signs of rats being in residence. Moving right along, we saw another apartment which was clean but again, far too small for our needs. Finally, late in the evening and after getting lost a few times, we arrived at the third apartment in the Hinjewadi area of Pune, an area central to the city's international IT hub. This apartment block, managed by a company called Hummingbird, was also the most expensive, but we knew instinctively even before going inside that we had hit the jackpot. Close to the apartment, we had passed many restaurants and hotels as well as a D Mart, one of the main grocery store chains in India. The complex was massive with blocks and blocks of apartments surrounding and overlooking a central golf course. Construction work was certainly still evident but more so in the distance than on the doorstep. The grounds of the complex were finished to a high standard. If we wanted, we could easily bring the babies out for a walk, for there were lots of communal areas with seating and walking tracks. There was also a swimming pool, small shop, gym, games room and table-tennis tables on-site. It was all looking good so far.

We went through the usual security check and headed for the manager's office located on the third floor. The building was very new and clean, and there seemed to be lots of comings and goings. People were bustling around the place, children were playing outside and a notably friendly atmosphere prevailed. The manager, Surendra Bisht, led us up to see the apartment on floor twenty-two. He was a young, efficient and friendly man who could display a broad smile at the drop of a hat. The apartment itself was fantastic, spotlessly clean, spacious and bright with a large balcony overlooking the golf course. There were two bedrooms, one with a shower en suite and loads of storage space. The second was big enough to store all the baby gear and our luggage. There was also a large separate bathroom with both shower and bath. The kitchen was basic but had what we needed: a microwave, fridge and kettle. We could rent a two-ring gas hob if we wanted, and there was loads of cutlery, crockery, cooking utensils, pots and pans. The sitting room was a large open-plan room with a dining area. It was well-furnished, spacious and had marble floors. Wi-Fi was included in the cost as was breakfast and daily cleaning. There was a communal dining room where breakfast was served. They could also provide us with dinner on a daily basis for a nominal charge of three euro per person. Suitably impressed, we wanted to take it immediately. However, Surendra needed to check if it was possible for us, as private tenants unaffiliated to any IT company, to rent the apartment. Apparently the apartments were usually leased to companies for use by their employees working in the nearby IT village. He assured us he would get back to us the next day. In the meantime, in order to speed up the process, we completed all the paperwork required before leaving, hoping against hope to be able to rent it.

Later that evening and wrecked from the long day apartment hunting, we marked my birthday by going out to dinner with Edel and Denise. The restaurant was recommended by Rajesh, and despite the worry of searching for an apartment as well as still having to buy all the baby equipment, we really had a lovely evening. Seán gave me a beautiful bracelet; one of the charms on it was of two babies intertwined.

We got the call the next evening confirming we could rent the apartment. It worked out at €45 per day, more expensive than we had budgeted for but it ticked all the boxes, and more importantly, we didn't have the time for any more searching. We needed to focus on getting the baby equipment; a crib, bottles, steriliser, formula and car seats being the most essential items. We decided it would be easier and more practical to buy the car seats when back in Mumbai, so at least we had two less items to think about. We had researched baby shops online and were heading to three different shopping malls in order to get the best prices. The cost of baby stuff was really no different to home. It was just that buying in India meant we didn't have to lug everything with us from Ireland. The downside was that products were not as modern as those at home, but that's the trade-off.

Later that evening, after we had unpacked all of our purchases, we went in search of Surendra to pay for the apartment for four weeks. We explained we were going back to Mumbai and told him when our approximate date of return to the apartment would be. We then went off to meet with Rajesh to break the news to him that we had found someplace else and would no longer be renting from Abhijeet. Rajesh knew the apartment was not suitable for us but probably hoped we would stick it out, but he hadn't bargained on the Malone–Whyte resolve. When we broke the news to him, he was OK about it but still asked if he could contact us when his own apartment became available. He felt we still might change our minds and want to move. We agreed to his request as we learnt the hard way that it's always good to have other options or at least a plan B. Returning to our new apartment in Hinjewadi that night to settle in, we had a good feeling. We both knew we wouldn't be moving anywhere else in Pune; it was perfect for us. At that moment in time it felt as good as home.

We ended up renting the two-ring gas hob so that we could cook ourselves. In hindsight, this was a mistake. We discovered it was difficult to buy any kind of meat in the supermarkets, and it was actually cheaper to eat out than to cook in. Beef is not available, and even though fish is sold in the markets, the flies swarming around it didn't exactly appeal to us. I searched the supermarkets high up and low down and still couldn't find any fish, but on one occasion I did manage to get what looked like chicken fillets. That evening we feasted on stir fried 'chicken' and rice. That was the first and last time we managed to purchase chicken, despite the daily sight of whole chickens hanging by their necks or feet in the small market stalls, which was not very appetising and not for the faint-hearted cook. We opted instead for the relative safety of the takeaway version.

Food in Indian restaurants, whether vegetarian or not, is delicious. Fish is available in abundance in India. Despite weird sounding names we had never heard before, it was always flavoursome and tastefully cooked. The Emerald Hotel was vegetarian. The food the restaurant produced was so delicious that I nearly contemplated becoming a vegetarian.

While the gas hob attached to the huge cylinder of gas sitting in the middle of the kitchen floor made me extremely nervous, I did manage to cook vegetarian fare a few times. I cooked rice and paneer cheese, a type of Indian cheese with a rich meaty texture. It's surprisingly tasty and something I have searched for in vain since returning to Ireland. In the end, and before I ended up a nervous wreck from checking and rechecking the hose and connectors insisting I could smell gas around the apartment, we gave up the ghost with the cooking bit. We had our dinner in the complex dining room or at local restaurants. Sometimes we ordered from the numerous takeaways, which for about €10 for the two of us was the cheapest and easiest way to satiate ourselves.

Seán, while he likes and eats most foods, could be described more so as a meat and two veg type of man. He is definitely not a fan of spicy food and was always careful in what he ordered. Towards the end of our stay in India, Seán didn't need to look at the menu. Instead, he had taken to pleading with the waiters for plain meat and 'spuds'. Surprisingly and most appreciated was the chicken and what looked like mashed potatoes that they obliged him with on several evenings. Still, Seán just couldn't wait to get home for Irish spuds, steak or bacon and cabbage. Mind you, it didn't help when our so-called friends at home were sending picture messages to us of plates laden with Irish stew.

During the first night in our new apartment, Seán had a domestic with the crib while trying to assemble it. Sweat dripped from him as he came to the conclusion that some of the pieces had to be missing. He couldn't be persuaded otherwise and according to him we'd have to return to the shop with it the following day. We asked Surendra for the loan of a screwdriver. He arrived a few minutes later and immediately set about helping to assemble the crib. Thank God for small mercies. He completed the job half an hour later and of course no pieces were missing. That was the nature of people in India; we found everyone to be friendly, courteous and helpful. We sat around and had a beer with him, and he asked about the babies in his own inimitable gentle way. He seemed genuinely interested in where we were from, what Ireland was like and about us and our babies. He made it easy for us to open up and tell him our story. He left shortly after midnight giving us his email address and phone number to keep in contact. He begged us to let him know how the birth went and whether we had boys or girls. That night we received the confirmation email from the clinic. The birth was scheduled for Thursday, and we must be at the hospital for 11 a.m. Given the excitement of the last few days and what we were going to face over the following days, that night, for the first time since we landed in India, we slept easy.

30

OUR SOLICITOR
IN MUMBAI

Although we had lost time searching for alternative accommodation, we were content and easy now knowing we had somewhere perfect to bring our babies back to. Leaving Pune at 6 a.m. the following morning in the hope that we would miss the worst of the traffic on our approach into Mumbai was wishful thinking on our part, for the roads were as congested and clogged as ever. After checking into the old reliable Emerald Hotel in Juhu, we met our solicitor and her husband who was also her business partner. Their office was located inside and at the rear of a large shopping mall called the Mega mall, which was bustling with crowds of shoppers.

The tiny office was within a warren of little alleys housing hundreds of tiny business units in the mall. The unit was so small you literally could not have swung a cat in it. To put it into context, our solicitor and her husband had to go into the room first to sit behind the desk. When positioned there, it was only then Seán and I could fit into the tiny space opposite the desk. Edel and Denise had to stand outside and film in through the glass window. We were offered the obligatory drink of tea or water and then we got down to business. They were a larger-than-life couple who seemed to work well together. They spoke very quickly in broken English with a strong accent. At times it was frustratingly difficult to understand them, most particularly her husband. They didn't seem to mind being asked numerous times to slow down or to repeat themselves, but then seconds later off they'd go again, at a hundred miles an hour.

They referred to their copy of the Irish Surrogacy Guidelines as they told us the process in India to get the emergency travel certificates. They outlined what was required of us and what was their responsibility as our solicitor. Reviewing the contract, they checked each page to ensure it was completed and signed correctly, commenting that it was a legal requirement in India to complete all sections of the contract in advance of the surrogacy process being initiated; otherwise the contract could be deemed invalid. They spotted the section of the contract which we had not completed in relation to who we appointed to care for our babies should we both die before they were born. At some point during our discussion, this section did a Houdini and disappeared from the contract.

They wrote down the steps in the process for us while going through each required document and outlined who was responsible for getting what done. Once our babies were born, we were to email them the following details:

- Our names in full and our address in Ireland.
- Our babies names in full.
- The sex of the babies and their date of birth.
- The height of the babies.
- The weight of the babies.
- Their time of birth.

We needed to register our babies while in hospital so that their birth certificates could be issued and then following receipt of the birth certificates we needed to arrange the DNA testing. It was also our responsibility to get documents for the FRRO including:

- A no-dues letter from the Corion Clinic.
- The process letter from the clinic.

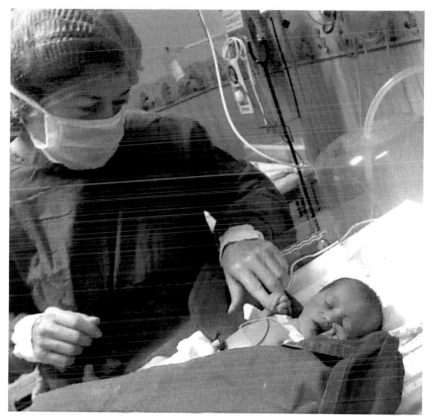

Visiting Donal in the Neonatal Intensive Care Unit, Dr L H Hiranandani Hospital, Mumbai, 26 September 2013.

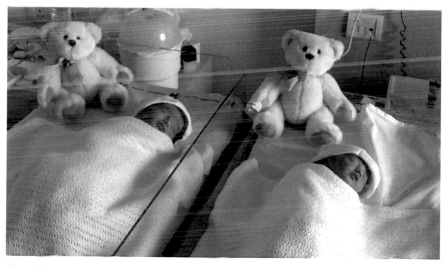

First day together, 29 September 2013.

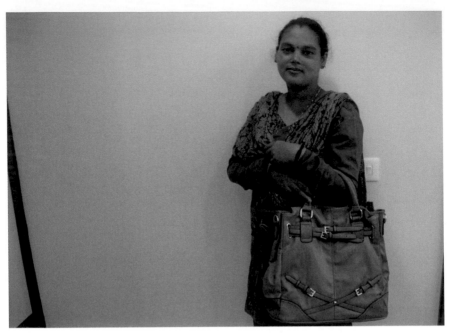

Shobha Dinesh Pandey, June 2013.

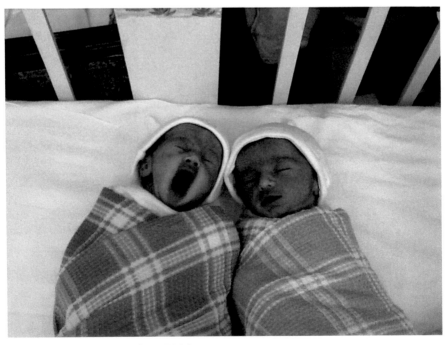

Ruby and Donal, October 2013.

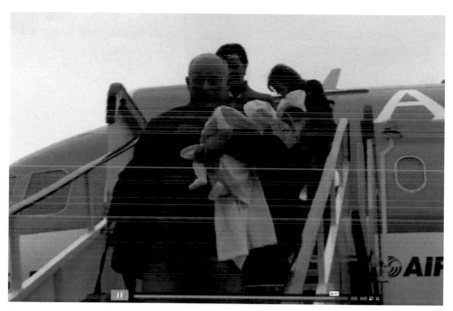

Home at last! Arriving at Shannon Airport, 9 November 2013.

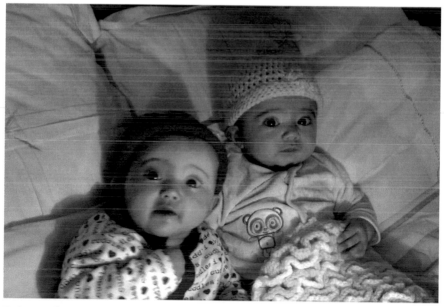

Ruby and Donal, March 2014.

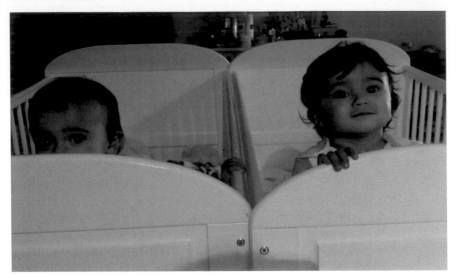

Ruby and Donal at home, November 2014.

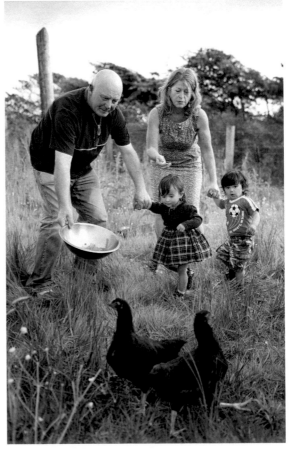

Seán, Fiona, Ruby and Donal at home, June 2015. Courtesy of Eamon Ward.

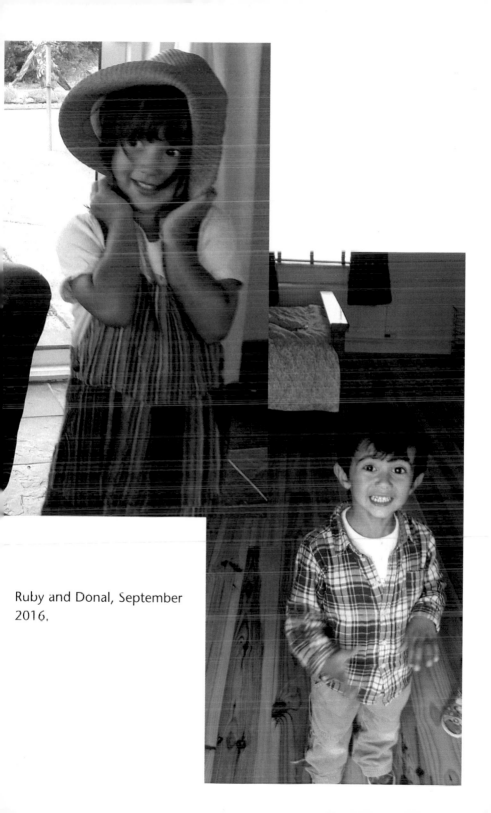

Ruby and Donal, September 2016.

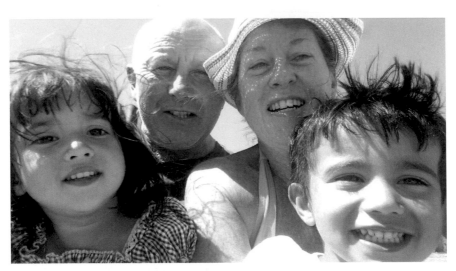

Ruby, Seán, Fiona and Donal, August 2016.

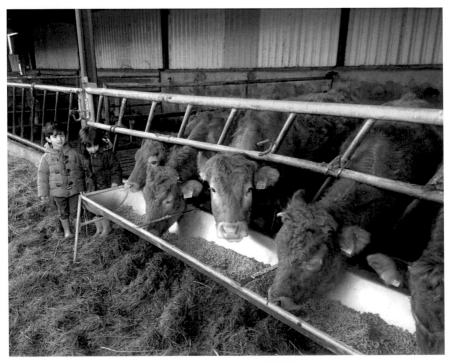

Donal and Ruby feeding the cows, January 2017.

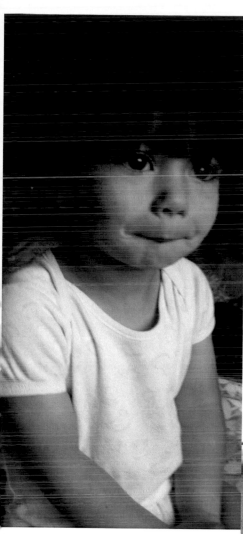

Ruby, October 2015.

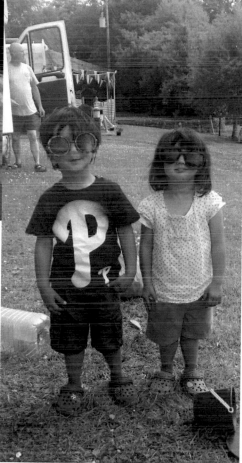

Donal and Ruby, June 2016.

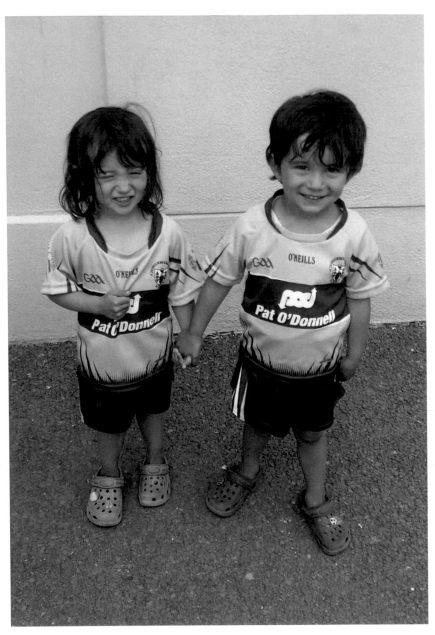

Up the Banner! Ruby and Donal proudly wearing their Clare jerseys, June 2016.

- A no-dues declaration from the hospital.
- 12 passport photographs of each baby.

Their responsibility included obtaining the following from the clinic:

- The pre-natal record.
- Cycle summary to include the date of treatment commencement.
- Doctors registration certificates.

They would then prepare all of the documents and affidavits required; four copies of each to include:

- Consent of Shobha and her husband to DNA testing.
- Affidavit of the doctor who collected the DNA samples.
- Affidavit of marital status of Shobha and her husband in both English and Hindi.
- Affidavit of our lawyer stating she had translated all documentation to Shobha and her husband.
- Affidavit from Shobha and her husband stating no objection to the issuing of travel certificates for our babies.
- Affidavit from Shobha and her husband stating they have no objection to us having sole custody and guardianship of our babies.
- The full address of Shobha and her husband so that they could be put on notice of legal proceedings.
- The contact details and email address of the Corion Clinic.

They took photocopies of our passports and we explained how we came to have tourist visas as opposed to medical visas. They told us that irrespective of the fact that the new Indian Visa Guidelines had come into effect after we had started the surrogacy process, we were still now required to comply with them. The first hurdle we needed to get over was the requirement to be married. They didn't bat an eyelid when we explained we weren't married, instead they explained we needed to get a declaration from our solicitor in Ireland stating that we had been cohabitating for whatever number of years and that as such we are to be considered a 'couple' in every sense. We were to be considered common-law husband and wife and this would suffice. There really was a way around everything in India.

As we discussed further the issue of the medical visa, explaining the reasons why we didn't apply for it, they interjected and said we would have had no problem getting a medical visa. They produced a copy of a letter that clearly stated Irish applicants seeking a medical visa for the purposes of surrogacy were to be accommodated in getting the visa. They were right. We would have got a medical visa no problem, but how were we to know this? We were left believing we were not eligible to even apply for a medical visa let alone that we would get one. It certainly wasn't for lack of trying; we had asked enough questions but still no one thought to tell us. There was no way out of this one. We would just have to proceed as it was and suffer the consequences. Hopefully, according to them, we would just get a fine and a rap on the knuckles for this breach. They were more confident than us in believing we could overcome this issue, but either way we had no choice except to keep moving forward and deal with it when we had to.

Seán mentioned about paying *chai-pani* (a bribe) to deal with this issue or to get things done quicker, but this was dismissed out of hand saying *chai-pani* was not accepted in India. We knew differently. We knew from the person who had gone before us that *chai-pani* was accepted and not only that, at times it was absolutely expected in India. We didn't argue and said no more deciding to keep our powder dry with that one, and if necessary we could chance offering *chai-pani* ourselves. We paid them Rs. 75,000 (€1,060) upfront for their services. This was the agreed set fee. Only something unforeseen would alter it. Seán counted out and handed over the money to her husband who was obviously the money maestro of the partnership. After we mentioned that we needed to get money changed, they arranged for a friend of theirs to come with rupees within the hour. They explained then that we could do the rest of our business over the phone, by email or courier service, and we would probably only need to meet once more when we returned to Mumbai in a few weeks' time.

Mothercare in India was the wake-up call, a bit of a reality check for us, to say the least. We were wandering around the shop looking at bits and pieces when we heard the sound of a baby crying loudly. Seán passed a comment about the sound effects being very realistic, when suddenly we rounded the corner of an aisle and came face-to-face with a dad trying to sooth a tiny baby in his arms. Jesus, they weren't sound effects at all. It was all ahead of us! Putting aside our moment of anxiety, we refocused on the task at hand: car seats. They stocked only very basic car seats, which would have to do, but their prices were akin to the newest models at home. In contrast to the markets and bazaars, the shops in India have fixed prices, but Seán, loving the art of haggling, couldn't resist the temptation to try out his skills asking for a deal on two. After repeatedly trying to tell Seán that the prices were fixed, the shop assistant relented and gave us what we thought at the time was a good deal. It turned out that he had misquoted the price in the first instance and we ended up paying what they were advertised. They'll catch you somehow.

It was almost lunchtime when we headed off to have a wander around Bandra, one of Mumbai's many markets and bazaars where the bantering and haggling is a way of life, an expected art form. Bandra is a bustling cauldron of stalls and hawkers selling everything and anything; if they don't have what you want there and then, they will get it for you. In India, there is nothing you can't get.

31

THE BIRTH DAY

Our babies were due to arrive into our world today. We checked out of the hotel after an early breakfast and took a couple of taxis to the hospital. Edel and Denise had arrived just ahead of us with the film equipment. Edel was going to try and film within the hospital, but we knew recording was not permitted. If taken to task on this, she was going to try to use our small camcorder discreetly, as if it were for personal purposes only.

Dr L H Hiranandani Hospital provides a variety of accommodation for families who wish to stay with their relatives while in hospital. We had booked a room in advance, as we wanted to make sure we had immediate access to our babies and that we could be with them and care for them as soon as possible. We had been told to go to reception on arrival and we would be directed to 'Client Relationship' for check in. We had also been told we could bring whatever baby supplies we needed for our stay, and that there was also a shop on-site where we could purchase other baby things if needed. This was where we had planned to buy the baby formula.

Following the security checks, we re-entered the hospital where we had been last January afraid to hope that we would be returning. The huge lobby area seemed even more crowded and daunting than it had previously. We took our turn in the queue to have our passports checked; then we were directed to another waiting area outside the 'Client Relationship' office to wait for the social worker who would go through the paperwork.

One important thing to remember about India is that an appointment time is meaningless. It is something that is given but is never ever adhered to. You will wait for hours to be seen, and there will never be an apology or reason given. It is as if you had turned up unannounced. It was frustrating at times. We had to come to the realisation that this was the way things were in India. We learned to take this into consideration even when ordering taxis or takeaway food, ordering a few hours in advance to when we actually wanted them. There was no point in getting annoyed or angry; it was not going to change the people or the system. Once this is accepted that sense of frustration dissipates and a state of acceptance prevails, at least where appointments are concerned anyway.

A slightly built man eventually emerged from 'Client Relationship' and ushered us into the small space he used as his office. We piled in with our mountain of luggage and baby equipment, afraid to leave it outside. Once inside, there was hardly room to shut the door behind us. He didn't bat an eyelid, so presumably he was used to people like us bringing the kitchen sink and all into his office. He sat across from us, rifled through stacks of papers, clicked on his computer and went back to rifling through papers, completely ignoring us. Meanwhile, we were wondering if Shobha was giving birth. Maybe our babies were already born while we were just sitting around being ignored. Seán was getting more and more agitated, particularly when the social worker kept facilitating numerous unannounced interruptions from people coming into his office to speak with him.

Finally he addressed us and from there on in proved to be both efficient and friendly. He started by checking the contract, then our passports and visas and the receipt for the advance payment to the hospital. As he checked them, he filled out some forms which we were asked to sign and duly did without a clue what they were about. Then he told us that we needed to wait until after the birth before checking in to our hospital room. We presumed this was in case something went wrong and there may be no room required. He announced he was going to bring us to the second-floor delivery suites and introduce us to Dr Anita Soni, the doctor who was going to deliver our babies. Dragging all our luggage behind us, we emerged from the lift into a large lobby adjacent to a small waiting room and once again we were checked by security. We had to remove our shoes and leave them at the entrance to the waiting room, which was filled with people, some sitting on chairs, some lying on the floor and some on seats not unlike futons. We were all there for the same reason – all expectant parents or relatives waiting on news of a birth.

We left our luggage in the care of Denise and walked quickly to the delivery theatres to be introduced to Dr Soni. Speaking briefly to us in English, she said she would be carrying out the caesarean section at about 12.30 p.m. and we should return to the waiting room until we were called. Back in the waiting room you could cut the air with a knife as the tension built up. Every time the door opened we looked expectantly to the person calling out the name, signalling to someone in the room that their new family member had arrived into the world. People leaned forward to hear what name was being called and then settled back again to wait, while the person fortunate enough to have the long wait over, hurried outside to meet their new arrival. And so we suffered the intolerable wait, getting more and more anxious as time moved on. One o'clock and no news; half past one and still nothing. By two o'clock the tension was increasing by the minute as we wondered if something had happened. Had something gone wrong? Seán glanced my way every so often and saw the look of worry etched on my face. Unable to read the paper any longer, my fingers tapped with anxiety and as a result, he was starting to feel edgy. Surely it didn't take that long to carry out a caesarean section? Something had to be wrong.

While waiting we reflected on our time with Edel and Denise. What we had expected to be a difficult time with a camera crew breathing down our necks was in fact quite the opposite. They had become friends during our journey, mucking in and helping us with everything from sourcing alternative accommodation to buying the baby stuff, as well as being good craic and great piss-takers. They were there when needed and offside when not. Overall, it was a comfort to have them on board while they were making the documentary but more especially there as our friends.

Eternity seemed to pass, not once but several times, until finally at 3.30 p.m. it was our turn to hear our names called. Denise stayed behind as we grabbed our shoes and scurried down the corridor towards the delivery rooms, followed by Edel carrying the camcorder. Standing outside the theatre, we strained to get a glimpse of our babies or even just to hear a cry. Two gowned and masked staff members were walking towards us, each holding a baby, literally each holding a baby in just one hand ... and we saw our babies for the first time.

We looked at each other speechless, and then our gazes shifted back again to our babies. We still didn't know for sure, no one had said anything. Were they really our babies? Were they OK? Were they boys or girls? Was Shobha OK? Dr Soni was suddenly in front of us flanked by the two staff holding 'our' babies.

Pointing to her right, she said, 'So this is the boy. He was lifted first and he weighs 2.3kg.' Then turning to her left, she said, 'And this is the girl. She weighs 2kg. They are fine.'

My God, through all the heartbreak and disappointment we had arrived in Mumbai to experience this on this day. Could there be any more happiness and joy in our lives?

32

DONAL & RUBY

Our miracles, Donal Fintan Malone and Ruby Darina Malone, have their birth time recorded as 2.41 p.m. with Donal first out followed closely by Ruby. I recall Seán saying some time later to me that the minute he saw them he instinctively knew, without indication, we had a boy and a girl. He doesn't know how or why but he just knew. My mother's prayers had been answered and our journey home to her would be somewhat easier for that. There was nothing between here and home now only paperwork.

Dr Soni wanted Donal to go to the Neonatal Intensive Care Unit (NICU) as she was concerned that he might have some fluid on his lungs which she could cause some breathing difficulties. Of course they were also going to take Ruby along for observation. For now we couldn't have them to hold. We would have to make do with just looking and longing. Dr Soni reassured us again that everything was OK, and it was more a matter of routine that they both go to NICU. We asked how Shobha was. For a split second, Dr Soni looked at us blankly, then quickly realising who Shobha was she replied brusquely that she was fine. She was abrupt almost like Shobha didn't matter, and her indifference stung us. Later and as we observed and interacted more with her, it became apparent that this characteristic was employed during every discussion or conversation with us, with staff, with anyone. It was an inherent characteristic synonymous with those who are in positions of power. Her attitude however couldn't dampen our elation as we walked away from our precious cargo, leaving them in her capable hands. Returning briefly to the waiting room to collect our belongings, those still waiting to see our beaming faces asked us what we had. They were genuinely so pleased and happy for us that it was humbling.

We returned to reception to check in to our room. With both Donal and Ruby now in NICU we could have gone to a nearby hotel, but we didn't want to be away from them, not for a second longer than we had to. We paid the room deposit and were given the standard welcome pack which contained the hospital brochure, a hospital pass to be presented every time we entered or exited the hospital and money-off coupons for services such as dental care should we wish to make use of them during our stay. We were then taken, along with our baggage, to our room on the eleventh floor. This floor catered only for parents and relatives of babies born through surrogacy such was the demand it seemed. Security personnel escorted us to our room after first checking our bags. If we needed to leave the floor or the hospital for any length of time, we had to inform the security guard who in turn was responsible for locking our room door after us and on return letting us back in again.

Turning left just past the large nurses' station we came to our room, number 1107, which was one of the basic room options available. We chose this room as opposed to a larger room or a suite simply because it was the cheapest at Rs. 5,500 (€78) per night. It had everything we needed: en-suite facilities with a single hospital-style bed and a large couch for sleeping, as well as a wardrobe, small dressing table and a TV. The room was bright and spacious enough for us and a large window provided panoramic views over the city. Tea and coffee making facilities were provided, and there was some space for luggage and baby equipment. Towels, sheets and all our meals were provided. Much to our surprise, the hospital food was very tasty and palatable. The nurse came in and showed us how to use the phone, TV and the call-bell system. At that moment in time, they could have housed us in a cowshed; we didn't care, we were running on adrenaline, elated. We texted and phoned everyone waiting at home for news. Over the previous few days and hours we had been receiving tons of texts from our friends and family eager for the news. It seemed everyone at home, like ourselves, had been waiting with bated breath.

We could visit NICU any time. So while Denise held the fort, Seán and I, followed by Edel with the camcorder, headed for the NICU back down on the second floor, the same floor as the delivery theatre. We were doubtful, but Edel hoped that maybe she would be able to get a couple of shots of us with our babies. Emerging from the lift, it was obvious the security guard recognised us as he smiled and shouted something to his colleague outside NICU. We presumed he told him who we were, as he opened the door for us to the NICU without questioning or searching us. Once inside the small waiting area, we rang the bell to alert the nurse to us. Edel was immediately banished, as only parents were allowed in to visit and only one at a time, so I went first while Seán and Edel remained outside. Before entering I had to remove my shoes and put on flip-flops. I was led into a small annex where I was required to remove all jewellery, wash my hands, put on a gown, hat and mask. Then I was brought in to spend my first moments with my son and daughter.

Swaddled tightly in white blankets with only their little faces peeping out, they were tiny but perfectly tiny. Swaddling babies is routine in India. It is a specific way of wrapping the baby tightly in a blanket to create a comfortable, safe and secure feeling, similar apparently to being in the womb. It is supposed to induce warm feelings and help the baby relax, sleep and feed. It's a lovely idea and was something we would continue for as long as possible. Donal was slightly darker in complexion and presented a mop of black hair, while poor petite Ruby was as bald as a coot, not a screed of hair. I had the iPad with me to take some photographs, but all that went completely out of my head as I just stood there gaping at them enthralled. I couldn't touch Donal who was inside the glass bubble of an incubator. He was rigged up to IV lines, and oxygen and feeding tubes were taped down into his little nose. As Ruby was only there for observation or more likely just to keep him company I was allowed to touch her. Stroking her little face, I talked to her, welcoming her to our world and telling her all about our family waiting at home and her brother in the next bed. The nurse returned and again reassured me that Donal was doing very well, and just to reaffirm this she lifted the cover of his incubator inviting me to touch him. Tentatively I reached out and stroked him with one finger, afraid I was going to hurt him. Strangely it was the bigger more robust fellow that was unwell and vulnerable now, while tiny Ruby was larger than life in the next bed. Exercising her lungs with gusto, she was certainly intent on letting us all know that she too had arrived. I talked to them for another while and then suddenly remembered I had the iPad and was meant to be taking some photographs. I managed to inadvertently get a short video clip before being reprimanded. Only photographs were allowed. In fairness, throughout our stay, the professionalism and efficiency of the hospital staff was incredibly reassuring at a time when we were so anxious and vulnerable. Eventually, before I would be accused of hogging all the time with our children, I skipped out on cloud nine to give Seán his long overdue turn.

Later that night, it wasn't the uncomfortably hospital bed, the small couch, the hot and stuffy room or the noise from the corridors that kept us awake, but thoughts of the two tiny beings that we had brought into the world, that were now our world.

At home in West Clare, and particularly unique to our area, there is a way of referring affectionately to people as 'the lads'. 'How's it going lads?' or 'what are ye up to lads?' can be heard daily around our area. So before Donal and Ruby were born, we were already referring to them as 'the lads' and we continued to do so now. Our last evening on our own together, we ran the gauntlet and rambled out for some dinner. Despite Juhu being considered a good area in Mumbai, it didn't compare with this area, Powai. Here, we could have been in any cosmopolitan city in the world: Barcelona, London, New York or central Dublin. There were no beggars and no people sleeping on the streets. As we walked from the hospital to the commercial centre, we could see that the street structure was well planned and lined with majestic and architecturally beautiful buildings. The commercial centre itself had many fine shops and designer outlets, not very interesting but not prohibitively expensive either. We did find a bazaar where we purchased our first baby-changing bag for a very reasonable price, once again negotiated by Seán. We then recognised a Chinese restaurant, part of a chain in India, and headed for it. Again, it was like walking into any Chinese restaurant in any major city as opposed to being in India, and once again the food was fabulous. We ate and drank for Ireland knowing that tomorrow would be the start of a very different life together.

33

GETTING ACQUAINTED

After a long and restless night, breakfast arrived at 6 a.m. and with that the nurse came in to tell us that Ruby would be transferred to our room that day. They still had some concerns about Donal and needed to continue observing and treating him in NICU. After waiting as long as we could to allow the staff in NICU enough time to finish their morning work and for Edel and Denise to arrive, we ventured downstairs to see the lads.

Donal was still rigged up to oxygen and various other tubes. The nurses had concerns that he had developed a blood-borne infection, as both his temperature and white-cell count were raised. As a result, they had started him on IV antibiotics. However, the good news was he was feeding normally and without the help of a tube, so there was some improvement. Because of the possible infection we weren't allowed touch him that day. My heart almost broke as I looked down at our frail and vulnerable baby. I didn't know if he could hear me at all, but I spoke gently to him through the bubble telling him his mammy and daddy were waiting for him to get well and that we loved him.

Ruby on the other hand was flying it and ready for the change of scenery our room would bring. While Seán went in to see Donal, they prepared Ruby to be transferred back with us, but first we had to complete the application forms for registration. These were really important because they would result in us getting Donal and Ruby's birth certificates issued by the

Municipal Corporation of Greater Mumbai. It was imperative that these forms be completed correctly in the first instance. This meant they had to be legible and clear, otherwise the registration and birth certificates could be delayed or worse still, they could be registered with incorrect names, something which could not be altered or corrected after the fact. Any information already given, such as our home address, had to be completed exactly the same. There could be no deviation from what was already provided. If the person responsible for registering the births could not read the form, they would not revert to us to clarify. Instead, they would enter in the birth register what they thought or assumed the names to be. For the most part it is safe to say that Seán doesn't write legibly, so I was tasked with completing the forms. Deliberately and precisely, I tried to complete the forms with the significant distraction of Seán, Edel and Denise chattering away beside me. Finally, the forms were completed; the first of many pieces of documentation to be completed over the coming weeks. I returned them to the nurse who checked that everything was signed where it should be. As we waited for Ruby to be wheeled out, Seán took the opportunity to phone our solicitor to tell her the registration forms were completed. She was going to do what she could to speed up the process for us, but we should expect it to take anywhere from eight to ten days for the birth certificates to be issued.

Princess Ruby emerged in her little incubator, and we headed for the lift, which always took forever to arrive, as it stopped on every floor going up and down. People peered curiously at us when we got in, first at Ruby then at each of us. The men seemed to look at Seán in wonderment and what must surely have been envy as they tried to figure out how he managed to have three women in tow! Back in our room, both of us just stood like eejits looking down at Ruby. Neither of us had the courage to pick her up until Edel gently prompted us, and then it was like flicking a switch as I lifted her out of the crib and into where she belonged … her mother's arms. I smelt her baby smell and was consumed by that overwhelming rush of love that a mother instinctively feels when she holds her baby for the first time. The feelings all came hurtling back to me. She whimpered, yawned and settled in my arms – perfect.

We spent the day getting acquainted with our new addition, who was stunningly beautiful and gorgeous in the opinion of her two totally biased parents. She was a cracker, and we relished doting over her. She was taking 20ml of feed every three hours and between feeding her, visiting Donal and learning again all about babies, the hours just flew by. We were shown how to swaddle Ruby. She seemed so content and settled, that we knew to continue swaddling was absolutely the right thing to do for as long as Donal and Ruby would allow us. We went through the day, nappy changing, making up bottles, feeding, washing and sterilising bottles while in between we managed to grab a bit of dinner and watch some Bollywood.

34

AN EMBASSY
WITHOUT EMPATHY

We made contact with the Diagnostic Clinic in Mumbai responsible for taking the DNA samples to see if there was any way that the samples could be taken while we were in the hospital, as opposed to travelling across the city to the clinic with two small babies in tow. I suppose we were concerned about Donal more so, given his condition and heightened vulnerability. We also wanted to ask if there was any way that the samples could be taken before we actually got the birth certificates, simply to expedite the whole process. We explained our circumstances to the doctor tasked with taking the samples; how both had been in NICU and how Donal still remained there. We also explained our intention to move to Pune after we were discharged. In fairness, the doctor, without any hesitation, agreed to travel to us to take the samples. However, she outlined a more immediate problem as the OQPS in Ireland had only sent out one sampling set as opposed to two. Testing could not be arranged until the second kit arrived at the clinic. We wondered how that error could have occurred, as the clinic in Ireland had been fully appraised that we were expecting twins. Anyway, we didn't have time to ponder this. We would have to contact the clinic to get the second kit sent as soon as possible. However, we still had to wait a few hours before we could phone because it was still the middle of the night in Ireland. When we got speaking to the staff they were all apologies and arranged to courier the second sample kit immediately, but because it was Friday, it would be at least Monday at the earliest before it would arrive.

We got back on to the Diagnostic Clinic in Mumbai to tell them that the sample kit was on its way, and they arranged to contact us as soon as they received it. The doctor also confirmed that if the sample pack arrived early enough on Monday, she would travel to the hospital the same day to take the samples as long as we could arrange for a witness from the Irish consulate to be in attendance. Delighted, we assured her we would get on to the consulate immediately to request to have someone on standby for Monday.

The representative from the Irish consulate in Mumbai was Indian and was lovely to deal with, as well as being exceptionally kind and accommodating. When we explained again our situation and asked if she would come to the hospital to witness the sampling, there was no hesitation in her agreeing to our request. We were on the pigs back as everything was beginning to fall into place, but this was short-lived.

The bombshell fell later that day by way of a phone call from the Irish embassy in New Delhi. Their representative was Irish and she told us in no uncertain terms that we had no right to make any arrangements for DNA sampling with the Irish consulate. She was adamant that the Irish consulate took their directives and orders from the Irish embassy only and not from us … mere Irish individuals. I explained to her how we had received an email from OQPS with the name and contact details of the doctor from the Diagnostic Clinic, telling us to go ahead and arrange the testing. We emphatically explained that we weren't giving orders or trying to go over anyone's head, we just did what we thought we were supposed to do. Apologising profusely, I explained our circumstances but to no avail. We had burnt our bridges and she was having none of it. Firstly she said we had to wait until the birth certificates were issued to us and that would probably take another week or so. Then when we got the birth certificates, we were to contact OQPS who would let the embassy know, and then she in turn would make the arrangements with both the Diagnostic Clinic and the Irish consulate for the samples to be taken. Then and only then would we be told when the testing would be carried out. There was absolutely no consideration given to our request. She would not accommodate the sampling to be taken at the hospital, even if we were still not discharged. She was insistent that we would have to travel to the clinic. She said she would inform the Diagnostic Clinic and the consulate of this current change in arrangements, and we were not to make contact with the Diagnostic Clinic or the consulate again.

I got off the phone from her despondent and fuming. I was enraged that we as Irish citizens could be treated with such contempt. The circumstances, which we genuinely felt to be extenuating, would not be entertained never mind considering what was in the best interest of the children. The embassy dictated how things were to be done, in what order and at what pace, irrespective of the fact that we were in a foreign country, alone, vulnerable and most importantly, we were Irish citizens whom they were supposed to support and help. Despite everyone else being more than willing to consider the welfare of the children and accommodate our request, the embassy downright refused to help us. It just seemed so ludicrous. When I explained to Seán what had happened, he phoned the embassy back to see if he could persuade them to consider the inhumanity of having to travel across the city for what would be a four-hour round trip in a taxi with two babies, but she was determined and would not change her mind.

It was still the rainy season, so at the drop of a hat the weather could change from searing heat to torrential rain quickly followed again by bursts of bright sunshine. Humidity was always high, so if you went outside for only a few minutes you ended up soaked with sweat. The only relief was to cool down with a cold shower. The view from the massive expanse of window in our room shimmered from the heat. It reminded me of the westerns I watched in my youth with cowboys trudging over dry land weakened from the lack of water and the arid desert heat. It was a magnificent view; our room was high enough to see all the way across the lake, over the city to the edge of the Arabian Sea. We welcomed this sight daily, living as we do beside the ocean at home.

This was Edel and Denise's last day in Mumbai before heading home, and we knew now they probably wouldn't get to meet Donal in person before leaving. We also knew we would miss them terribly because as well as being a great help and support to us, they were also our friends and only support while here. Donal was remaining in NICU on IV antibiotics for yet another day, as the doctor was still concerned about the lingering infection. We took each day as it came, hoping that he would improve sufficiently to allow him to be transferred to us, maybe even before Edel and Denise had to leave for the airport. Generally only relatives are allowed visit within the hospital, so every day Edel and Denise were 'our relatives'. The holdall bag they carried with them everywhere contained the camera hidden from view beneath clothes. Every day they took a chance as their bags were scanned coming into the hospital, but they were never questioned about it. During any filming we always locked the bedroom door in case someone entered unexpectedly; we couldn't take a chance on getting caught. Anytime someone tried the door there was a scurry to hide the camera, which was usually behind the couch. We justified these actions because we believed this recording would allow viewers to see what we were experiencing while in hospital. It was not for any other dishonest or deceitful purpose. The staff had no problem with us taking photos; it was filming they had an issue with.

During the days, we passed some time by taking turns going to D Mart just down the road for supplies. If it was raining, a rickshaw could be got outside the hospital for only €1.50, a pittance, and if sunny then the short walk down was a welcome ramble. Today was flying by and it was Seán's turn to do the shopping. On the list today were biscuits, milk, coffee, chocolate, nappies and wipes. He also chanced buying two cans of beer in the full knowledge that he would be searched coming back in, and they probably would be confiscated. He was and they weren't. We relished and thoroughly enjoyed this unexpected treat with dinner that night. Television wasn't much good to us, as the only English-speaking channel was CNN news, repeating the same headlines several times a day. The alternative was to watch Bollywood films. Mumbai houses India's Hindi film industry or as it is better known, Bollywood. Everyone seemed to adore watching these films. Everywhere you go there are giant posters on display advertising the latest Bollywood blockbuster, and in restaurants and every other public place, huge TV screens adorn the walls airing the latest over-acted Bollywood film. Apparently in Mumbai, there are over a thousand Bollywood films churned out annually, even more than Hollywood.

35

ALL-IRELAND DAY

The laptop lay opened but idle. We were unable to get a Wi-Fi connection because we hadn't applied in advance at the nurse's station, where the request would be referred to the hospital IT department to establish the connection and issue a password. Like everything else, the process could take hours and in our case days, even in this great nation known for its progressive technology. Another call was logged with the IT support department. We needed the internet connection not only to send emails, but more importantly, to access the All-Ireland Hurling Final replay between Clare and Cork. We had been to the final a couple of weeks previous in Croke Park. We only came away with a draw and now it was show time again. Seán would lose his reason if he couldn't see or at least hear the game. Just in case all else failed, Seán's sister Marion had been given instructions to record the game and post the disc onto us, including of course the hours of compulsory post-match analysis. Meanwhile, we hoped the IT department would resolve the problem.

Because of the time difference throw-in was at 8 p.m. in India, so we still had some time to get things sorted. But as the evening drew in and the throw-in got closer, Seán was getting anxious and repeatedly visited the nurses' station trying to get someone to sort out the problem. He was pacing up and down, anxiously checking the clock every five minutes. Hurling is in Seán's blood. He grew up steeped in the game and believes there is no other game on the planet that can touch the skill, pace and excitement of hurling. Couple this with the fact that Clare didn't get too many chances of winning an All-Ireland, and you can imagine how important watching this game was.

Right on cue, someone from customer service paid us a visit looking for feedback on hospital services and facilities. We said the food was great, but we needed an internet connection. The hygiene and cleanliness was up to standard, but we needed Wi-Fi. The staff were prompt in responding to our needs; they were wonderful, except when it came to sorting out the internet. Just as she attempted to ask another question, Seán halted her in her tracks and said, imploringly, 'It's nearly throw-in time. Please! We need the internet now.' She smiled calmly and agreed to sort everything out on Monday. Ah, customer service.

The only option was for one of us to go to the shared sitting room with the laptop and try to connect to the hospital Wi-Fi. Off I hurried to check it out. I got connected but I couldn't get the station up to watch the game. However, I could get a radio broadcast from Clare FM. It was the best that could be done and Seán would at least get to hear the game live. The build-up to the game was in full swing as he raced to the sitting room located directly across from the nurse's stations. During the game Seán's antics could be seen clearly by the nurses and I knew they were in for some treat. Luckily there was no one else trying to relax in the sitting room, divine intervention or sheer good luck on their part.

It was an absolute nail-biter. Every now and again Seán raced up to the room to update me. I just couldn't imagine what the nurses were thinking as he rubbed his head in frustration, cursed, paced up and down and inevitably shouted at the screen. With only eight minutes to go, the audio crashed. Seán was in an awful state pleading with me to get the sound back, but try as I might I couldn't get it working. The staff weren't at all happy with this unexpected turn of events either, judging by the large gathering around the nurses' station enjoying Seán's performance throughout. I returned to the room to break the bad news and found Seán getting a blow-by-blow account of the game via texts from David and Donal, right up to the end of the game when Clare was triumphant. The nurses heard the Clare roar for the first time that evening and witnessed Clare hurling mania first-hand. While we would have loved to have been there, we celebrated quietly instead, hoping for next year with Donal and Ruby in tow.

36

JUGGLING BABIES & BUREAUCRACY

We were awakened at cock-shout by cleaners and nurses bustling in and out of the room, and breakfast arrived shortly afterwards. We ate very little. We were tired from being up half the night, talking about the game and tending to our daughter. Ruby was sleeping, so we managed to doze off again only to be woken by Edel and Denise coming to say goodbye. It was a pity they hadn't yet met Donal in person. They would have to wait until we were back in Ireland for the privilege.

Just before lunch, Donal made his entrance. Now with both of them lying side by side, we examined them in turn, looking for the similarities that we expected to see in twins as well as any likeness to Seán. Donal still looked thinner and frailer, but he was also longer and slightly darker than Ruby. He had a head of shiny black hair, whereas Ruby was as bald as her dad. That was the only likeness there was. Something which we expected, but in reality was still strange to us, was their sallow complexions. Apart from that, they looked very different from each other.

It's very difficult to explain how very surreal that time was with unspoken questions fighting a battle in our heads and hearts. Would we love them immediately? Maybe we would have to learn to love them. Would we bond easily with them or would that happen with time? Obviously there is a worry that when you don't actually carry a baby for nine months maybe it becomes more difficult to love or to bond with? The immediate separation, particularly the longer separation from Donal, magnified that worry. These were very real anxieties, but as I looked down on them I felt again that intense instinct, that need to protect and care for these beings. Whatever the feeling I felt within me, it was tangible and consuming. They were our children, created by us in our love for each other and they were totally loved by us.

Then the here and now took over. The impact of having two beings was 'double trouble' and double the work. Ruby had just finished feeding before Donal arrived. He had been fed just before leaving the NICU, so they were OK for a couple more hours when we hoped we could start feeding them at the same time. Over the next while, we set about establishing a routine, taking turns washing, feeding and changing each of them in turn, marvelling in their being. We were intent on getting that routine going; otherwise, we knew we'd be all over the place and end up exhausted and wrecked. We watched in amazement as they seemed to connect with each other despite having been apart for a few days. They turned their heads towards each other almost as if they could smell each other or recognise the sound of each other's whimpers.

They were both on different formulas, something we hadn't thought about or planned for. Donal was on a high-calorie one while Ruby was on a regular type. This made life a bit more difficult, as it meant we had to be really careful not to get the bottles mixed up. On hindsight, we should have had different bottles for each one irrespective of formula. To simplify things now and make life easier, we bought another bottle type in the hospital shop. As with all newborns, feeding at this early stage took a long time. We took turns feeding each of them, so they would get used to both of us. Even at such an early stage, they seemed to be slipping into a routine together as they both settled into sleeping and feeding at the same time. During the night it was particularly difficult. We had been so used to uninterrupted sleep for so long, and now suddenly we were being woken up at all hours. Sometimes it took up to two hours before we'd be finished feeding and nappy changing. Our tiredness was compounded by nurses coming in at various times to check Donal's blood sugars and his temperature. Sometimes it felt we had only gone to sleep when breakfast arrived at the unearthly hour of 6.30 a.m. Later that same day we had a visit from Dr Soni, who advised us to increase the concentrate of both feeds to 40ml of water and one scoop of feed and to give a feed of 30ml each. They seemed to be improving in leaps and bounds.

There was a tinge of sadness in the middle of all this when Seán got a text message from Mairéad telling him that Thomas Downes had passed away. Thomas was a long-time friend of Seán's and had been unwell for some time. He was naturally upset and spoke of Thomas being a 'walking gentleman, full of life, fun and devilment'. He was convinced Thomas had held onto life to witness Clare beat Cork in the All-Ireland hurling final. I know Seán will miss him awfully.

The call came from the DNA Diagnostic Clinic the next day, informing us that the second sample kit had arrived. We could now contact the embassy to arrange the test for us. Hot on the heels of that call we received another, this time from the Irish consulate confirming that their witness was en route to the hospital to witness the DNA sample taking. Unfortunately and altogether too late, we realised that the consulate had never been informed by the embassy that the test had been cancelled. Feeling really bad about this, we had to explain about the embassy's refusal to allow us to have the test carried out in the hospital, and that they had said they would inform the consulate of the change of plan. Now this person from the consulate was sitting in a taxi in chaotic traffic probably for most of her working day. We didn't have any explanation as to why the embassy hadn't informed the consulate, but to us it was either a deliberate act or yet another example of inept bureaucracy, somewhat all the more worrying for us going forward. By way of distraction Dr Soni arrived to examine Ruby and Donal. Everything was fine and we could go home the next day. At least there was one piece of good news that day.

One of the nurses was arranging for the photographer to come and take the passport photos of Donal and Ruby for the legal paperwork. We needed twelve copies of each. The difficult part, it seemed, would be getting the snap with their eyes open. Later that morning the photographer arrived. He was a slight and quietly spoken young man with a state-of-the-art digital camera. Despite not speaking any English, he knew what was required and set to work. It only took him three minutes to photograph Donal with his eyes open, but Ruby took forever. She stretched, yawned and preened until finally, after about thirty minutes, she felt she was ready to pose and have her photo taken. We paid him Rs. 900 (€12) and he returned an hour later. However, he only had eight copies of each. Apparently they come in strips of eight as opposed to twelve, so off he went again to return an hour later with another strip. Thankfully, that was another job ticked off our to-do list.

While waiting for the birth certificates to arrive and the DNA tests to be done, we had two options to muse over. When discharged, we could go directly to Pune and then travel back to Mumbai with the lads to have the DNA test done, or stay on in Mumbai until the birth certificates were issued and the test done and then travel on to Pune. The latter appealed to us because we didn't want to do a round trip of over seven hours in generally unsafe driving conditions with Donal and Ruby. It meant paying for the apartment as well as a hotel in Mumbai, but we felt this was the better option and we hoped it would only be for a few days. We returned, yet again, to the tiny room and limited facilities at the Emerald Hotel, but with one additional and very important request: we needed a cot in our room.

We wanted to stock up on provisions before being discharged, so I headed down to D Mart, for nappies, wipes, formula and other bits and bobs. While browsing, I spotted some blankets perfect for swaddling the lads. I rambled slowly back up to the hospital in the searing heat with a rucksack full of baby supplies. I knew it was the last time I would do this walk, and I felt apprehensive at the thought of heading off into the sunset on our own with our small charges. As we packed for our reluctant release, I felt the need to take the cot sheets that the lads were lying on, as keepsakes for Donal and Ruby. They had the hospital crest and so would be another item for their memory box in time to come.

37

MEETING SHOBHA AGAIN

We talked a lot about Shobha: what she had done for us, how she had made it possible for us to have Donal and Ruby and what she had sacrificed for her family. We wondered if she was OK. We needed to know she was, but we were not permitted to visit her. The policy of the clinic and the hospital was that intended parents were not allowed to see the surrogate mother once she was admitted to hospital. During the pregnancy I had sent gifts to Shobha, for herself and her family, so before going out this time, I bought some gifts to bring with me, in the hope that we might get to see her. If not, I always had the option of leaving them at the clinic for her, but the problem with that was we didn't know if she would ever visit the clinic again. We felt she was probably still in the hospital given that she had a section, but we didn't know for sure. We decided to find out if she was still in hospital and if so which ward.

With my bag of gifts under my arm, I went to reception on the ground floor to ask if Shobha Dinesh Pandey was still an inpatient. The receptionist confirmed that she was and even more surprisingly told me she was in room 105 on the fifth floor. I thanked her and headed straight for the fifth floor. I tried to figure out how I was going to handle being stopped and questioned by security. The worst that could happen was I would be turned away. We had worked out that the general layout on each floor was the same, so I had a rough idea where the bedrooms were located and where security would be. As the lift came to a halt, I tried to look casual, took a deep breath and headed straight for the double doors leading to the ward. For all intents and purposes, I looked as if I did this trip every day. I was hoping to escape scrutiny by looking as if I knew exactly where I was going. However, the stern-looking security man stepped towards me and said something in Hindi. I smiled at him and kept going while at the same time pointing towards the bedrooms. He didn't shout, but he raised his voice authoritatively behind me, stopping me in my tracks. The game was up. As casually as I could muster, I turned smiling at him and said, 'I'm visiting Shobha Pandey in 105', and then I turned back nonchalantly and continued walking towards the doors. With my heart pounding in my ears, I listened for his voice again or worse his footsteps behind me, but nothing happened. Just as quick, I was through the doors walking towards the nurses' station. I glanced back half expecting to see him hurrying towards me ready to evict, but nothing, the doors were swinging closed.

Still not out of the woods, I saw a number of nurses busy working and writing at the station. Would they stop me or question me? Staring straight ahead, I continued on towards the rooms. As I passed the station, some of the nurses glanced up curiously. This was more about how I looked than anything else. I guess if you get through security you're considered legit because no one stopped me or asked me who I was or where I was going. It had been all too easy really for me to breach security, and that was a sobering thought given the level of security there was supposed to be in place throughout India. Beyond the desk, I turned left hoping to God the layout was the same on each floor. I couldn't risk wandering around searching for the room. That would definitely arouse suspicions. But sure enough there were the bedrooms and straight ahead was room 105.

The door was slightly ajar. I knocked quietly and gently pushed it open. It was a large enough room with two single beds. The bed nearest the door was empty but in the bed farthest away, beside the window, someone was lying with their back to me hidden from sight by the covers. I whispered 'hello', and as the form moved under the covers and began to turn towards me I realised my heart was still pounding. I recognised Shobha immediately. She sat up as I smiled and whispered 'hello' again, moving closer to the bed to get a better look at her. She looked tired and drawn, but she smiled in recognition and I felt reassured enough to sit and pull a chair towards the bed. Automatically I asked her in English how she was while pointing at her stomach. She couldn't understand me but intuitively she seemed to know what I was asking. She screwed up her face while pointing to her stomach and then her heart. Her face was as open as a book, telling me that she was hurting. She held her arms as if holding a baby and rocked them to ask me how Donal and Ruby were. I smiled and nodded in reassurance that they were fine. I didn't want to cry but tears were close. I didn't know what else to say; there was nothing I could say.

Someone was at the door. One of the nurses had come in to check on Shobha, and they spoke briefly in Hindi. I expected to be asked to leave or at the very least I expected to be questioned, but the nurse just turned to leave the room. I seized the opportunity and asked if she spoke English, to which she turned back and nodded saying she spoke a little English. I asked if she would give us a few moments of her time to translate for us. She nodded again and stood at the end of the bed. Shobha told me her stomach was very sore but they were giving her medicine for the pain. She said she was happy that our babies were born and were healthy. She asked if we were happy, and I told her we couldn't thank her enough. I told her our babies were doing really well and that we were due to be discharged the next day. I said how happy we were and how grateful we were to her. I told her we had named them Donal and Ruby, but omitted the fact that we had considered Shobha if we had a girl. Instead I asked her if she needed anything, anything at all. She shook her head. She didn't need anything, and she was being looked after by the staff. Her family had been in to see her and she was looking forward to going home to them, hopefully later in the week. Not really knowing why, I asked her if she would give me her address. Without hesitation, she wrote it down.

I haven't contacted Shobha and I really don't know if I ever will, but I think of the future and I want it for Donal and Ruby in case they ever want to meet her. If they do and we are alive, we will support and help them to find her. Time was up, and the nurse made a gesture for me to leave. Before I could move, Shobha took out her phone and took some photographs of me. Then as I stood and moved awkwardly towards Shobha, unsure of myself now, she opened her arms to me and we held each other silently in understanding. We would never see each other again. I didn't hand her the gifts, instead I just left them beside the bed. They were nothing compared to the gifts she had given us. Walking towards the door, I looked back one last time and then the tears flowed.

38

DISCHARGED

It was the first day of October, and after yet another early morning breakfast of omelettes and rice, we fed the lads. Donal only took 30ml while the guzzler Ruby Malone took a whopping 45ml. Today was the day we were to be let off out on our own to look after Donal and Ruby. This both excited and panicked us. Exhaustion won, however, and we fell back to sleep, only awakening at 8.45 a.m. to the sounds of the lads crying for their bottle. Seán, snoring loudly on the makeshift bed, was totally oblivious to their needs, obviously still exhausted. We knew we could hire a nurse or a nanny privately at any stage to help us. Before the lads were born, we had considered doing this even while we were in hospital, but we hadn't thought much about it after they arrived. Instead, we had just gone with the flow and managed away ourselves. It was always an option if we found things becoming too difficult or exhausting, so before leaving we got the number for Angels Agency in Pune from the hospital.

A junior doctor came in to check out the lads and commented that Donal looked a little jaundiced, but at the same time he said it was nothing out of the ordinary. The nurses then weighed the lads; they were back to their birth weight which was great. They also removed the 'cricket bat' from Donal's arm. This was a splint which had been placed under his arm to keep it straight while the IV cannula was inserted for administering the medications. We had christened it the 'cricket bat', quite an appropriate name given India's love of cricket. They gave us a supply of vitamins for Donal as well as a prescription for more and provided us with all the babies' medical reports, explaining everything in detail to us. Dr Soni arrived and asked if we were happy to be discharged that day, and as we nodded vigorously she gave us the all-clear to go. We were to visit her clinic in the Out Patient Department (OPD) before we left the hospital so that she could do a full check-up on the lads and to give us their record books for continuity when we returned home. She also wanted us to return to the OPD on the following Thursday or Friday between 9 and 11 a.m. for another check-up. We had the freedom to choose whichever day and time suited us to attend.

As we prepared to leave the hospital, Seán got a surprise phone call from our solicitor, telling us that she had the birth certificates and was couriering them to us at the hospital. We would have them in about forty-five minutes. We would get six original copies of the birth certificates, which was standard in India. There would be no means to get additional birth certificates again, so they needed to be carefully minded. We were amazed. It was barely five days since we had completed the registration forms, and we had the birth certificates already. We had been told it normally took eight to ten days, so we couldn't believe it. She must have used her influence, as she probably knew it would reflect well in the documentary. We didn't care what the motives were, we had them and we just relished in our good fortune. Maybe things were finally starting to go right for us. Seán was really hoping if we got the emergency travel certificates sorted quickly, we could maybe relax with a bit of down time and enjoy India before we were scheduled to fly home. I immediately got onto OQPS to tell them we would have the birth certificates shortly and requested they arrange with the Irish embassy for the DNA tests to be done as soon as possible.

While waiting outside the OPD clinic, we met a German couple and a Norwegian guy who also had babies born through surrogacy. It was becoming evident that surrogacy was a lot more prevalent than we had initially thought. The Germans told us that there were five babies born the previous night all through surrogacy, and in the queue that day waiting for check-up's and vaccinations prior to discharge, there were also five couples with babies all born through surrogacy. Obviously surrogacy was happening on a huge scale in India alone, and many people, not only from Ireland, were availing of surrogacy abroad. We were next in line. The lads were stripped of their layers, weighed again, had their heads and length measured, and all details were recorded in their books. We were then asked if we would like them to receive their vaccinations for BCG, hepatitis and polio before being discharged, and again we agreed. They were as good as gold through all the poking, prodding and needles. When finished, we went off with our discharge letter from Dr Soni to present to accounts in order to get our final bill.

During the course of our stay, we had been getting daily hospital bills itemising the charges in detail, and now we were given the final bill for our stay. Every single thing was itemised and charged to us, right down to the last nappy used. Of course there was absolutely no way of knowing if we had used all that was listed. Once our bill was settled we would get the letter we needed stating we had paid all our dues and nothing was owed. This would allow us to leave the hospital and apply for our exit visas when the time came. We had to present this letter to security when leaving, otherwise we wouldn't be allowed to go, simple as that. In the accounts department, we were told that we could only partly pay our bill, as Shobha was still an inpatient. We would have to wait for her to be discharged to settle her final bill. In the meantime, we had an interim letter permitting us to leave the hospital, but in order to get the no-dues letter we needed for our exit visas, we would have to return after Shobha was discharged on Thursday to finalise the bill. This fitted in with our plans, as we had to return anyway for the lads' check-up. Prior to our arrival in India we had transferred Rs. 100,000 (€1,410) as an advance payment to the hospital. On admission we paid another Rs. 25,000 (€352) and now we paid another

Rs. 132,000 (€1,862). We would have more to pay when we returned on Friday.

On the way back to our room, we bought sweets and chocolates for the nurses. This wasn't in any way adequate to express our gratitude for their professionalism, kindness and competence in supporting us during our stay and particularly for having to put up with our antics on All-Ireland day. Leaving our room for the last time, we thanked everyone including our diligent security man who had a broad smile plastered on his face as he waved goodbye. Maybe he was just delighted to see the back of the mad Irish couple. We trooped in to the foyer downstairs to wait for the birth certificates to arrive before getting a taxi to the hotel. Seán went off in search of a taxi big enough to take all of us along with the luggage, while I stood guard over the lads.

He returned at the same time as the courier arrived, amazingly exactly forty-five minutes after speaking to the solicitor. We set about checking the certificates to make sure there were no errors. We needed to make sure everything was correct and in order before we made the call to the embassy. There was a mistake. On one of the birth certificates one part of our address was spelled incorrectly. As is known in rural Ireland, addresses can be quite ambiguous, often with no house name, number or street, only the area or townland might be included. Our solicitor had advised us to give as much information and detail as possible regarding our address, so while 'Ballard Road' was not part of our address we included it to provide that additional detail and accuracy. Now we saw that on one certificate it was spelled 'Ballard Road' while on the other it was spelled 'Bellard Road'. We didn't know if this would cause any problems when we went to seek the emergency travel certificates or the exit visas, so before contacting the embassy, Seán phoned the solicitor for advice. She reassured us that this error was minor and should not cause a problem. Our next call then was to the embassy to request arrangements be made for the DNA testing.

Seán went out to ask the taxi guy to drive into the pickup area just outside the hospital. As he was walking back towards the door he reached for his phone, and even from a distance I could see he wasn't happy. Back inside he started reading out word for word exactly what was on the birth certificates to whomever was on the phone. After about ten minutes of this and more arguing he finished the call. OQPS were actually questioning if we had the birth certificates at all and wanted to know how we had got them so quickly. They actually did not believe we had the birth certificates. They had asked Seán to verify the stamp and signature on them, which he did, and still they did not believe we had them. It beggared belief. They demanded to know what we had done to get them issued so quickly, the implication being that we had done something illegal. When I had phoned them earlier to tell them we were getting the certificates, they hadn't raised any of these questions, so why now? Was it because the embassy made an issue out of it when OQPS had contacted them? Either way they did not believe us and refused to arrange the DNA testing until we scanned the birth certificates and emailed them to OQPS to prove they were in our possession. We found ourselves up against the clock. Someone out there was intent on making life excruciatingly difficult for us.

Our taxi was still waiting patiently for us, and once the price was negotiated we clambered in. The next problem was the seat belts didn't fit around the car seats; they were too short to go all the way around. We would have to get another taxi, but they were all the same. So I sat in the back between the car seats with an arm around each one trying to keep them steady, hoping the taxi driver would drive carefully. For all of my worrying he was an exceptionally careful driver, repeatedly checking to see if we were OK. The journey would take anything up to and probably over two hours given his careful driving. The air conditioning provided respite from the heat, but the glare of the sun through the glass was still very uncomfortable. To prevent the glare of the sun reaching their faces, I draped some muslin cloths over the car seats, and the lads slept soundly despite the bumpy conditions and continuous noise of car horns. En route, Dr Kadam phoned to tell us the documentation we required from the clinic for the legal process was ready for collection; namely their no-dues letter and a letter outlining the surrogacy process we had undertaken. Seán made an appointment to be at the clinic at midday the next day to collect the documents, and he was instructed to bring the original contract with him for verification purposes.

While we were stopped at yet another set of traffic lights, we were approached by an old woman begging. A common enough sight you might say. She looked about 70 years old, but most likely the years had not been kind to her and in reality she was probably only about forty. Tap-tap-tap went her frail hands on the glass as she moved around the car from window to window, smiling through gapped teeth and seeking eye contact. She stopped suddenly at one of the back windows when she noticed me straightening the cloth over Donal's seat. She had realised that there was not one but two babies in the car. I glanced up as the tapping became louder and more vigorous. Her hands were joined together in a pleading gesture, not for money but to see them. She just wanted to see our babies. She was missing most of the fingers from her right hand, and I wondered if she was one of those maimed deliberately as a child to attract more attention and pity when begging. I removed the cloths so she could see Donal and Ruby. She whooped loudly showing us what was left of her blackened teeth. She went from window to window, smiling and peering in at them, waving what fingers she had left and putting her hands together as if in thanks or in prayer. She had forgotten she was begging as she delighted in Donal and Ruby's presence. She was utterly enthralled with them. In India, it's tradition not to take babies out for at least the first three months of life. As a result, people are not used to seeing such young babies out in public.

The taxi began to edge forward. She tapped once again to catch my attention, and I saw she was blowing kisses at us. I quickly cranked down the window and practically threw her the notes I had been holding in my hand to pay the taxi driver. From the front, the driver shouted at me. I pretended not to understand his ire, but I knew full well he was furious because my actions would entice many more around the car. I didn't care and anyway we were moving slowing forward now. I looked at her as she walked beside the car. She moved slowly at first then quicker as she tried to keep up, and just as suddenly she stopped. We left her behind. I looked back to see her still standing between the fast-moving traffic, still smiling and still blowing kisses. The simplicity of showing love moved me. This vivid memory has remained with me long after many others have faded. I can only marvel at the ability of innocent babies to wipe a lifetime of hardship and pain from a face, even if only fleetingly.

Once again we were back at our Emerald Hotel, being greeted by the staff we had come to know so well. This time, however, all they wanted to do was look at Donal and Ruby; the lads were the centre of attention. Our small room was all prepared for us with a cot set up in a corner. Although well-used and a bit tired looking, the cot was spotlessly clean and had been very carefully made up. Sheets had been rolled up tightly into makeshift cot bumpers. Like most hotels, the Emerald offered free Wi-Fi access in the lobby and other public areas. However, it was at an additional cost in the bedrooms. We decided to pay for Wi-Fi because we couldn't be running up and down the stairs now. Unfortunately, just like in the hospital, there was a fault in our room and we had to wait for IT to fix it. We would have to traipse down to the lobby for a while. First things first, the lads were not willing to wait any longer for lunch, so as we fed them we caught up the news on television. We had lost touch with the outside world over the last few days; the headlines were all about the 'US Shutdown', whatever that was about.

Once we had them fed and settled, I went to get the birth certificates scanned and emailed to us, still frustrated this was even necessary. As I turned to go out the door, Ruby cried. I looked down at them both and realised this was what it was all about; however long things took didn't matter because everything was worth it for them. I closed the door gently, careful not to wake Seán who was catching forty winks on the bed. Reception informed me there was no access for guests to a printer or scanner, so I had to ask the staff to scan and email the birth certificates to me. The staff had no problem doing this ... once they got a quiet moment. There were three staff behind the desk and only myself in the lobby, yet another example of the frustratingly slow pace in India when trying to get something done. For the next couple of hours I wandered up and down the stairs checking and waiting on the email to come through, resisting the temptation to pester. It was over two arduously long hours later when my inbox finally received the scanned birth certificates, and I could forward them to OQPS. But by then, back in Ireland, it was after hours and offices were closed. It was now too late to request the DNA test be done the following day, which for us meant another frustrating delay. Delays, delays, nothing but delays.

39

DNA-TESTING
DIFFICULTIES

Time was moving on and it was now Wednesday, 2 October. We had to keep the pressure on to get the DNA samples taken soon. What time we had gained by getting the birth certificates earlier than expected was now lost because of OQPS and the embassy. The longer we were delayed the more expensive it was on us, as we continued to pay for both the hotel in Mumbai and the apartment in Pune. We couldn't afford to do that for too much longer. OQPS confirmed that they had received the scanned copies of the birth certificates but no other comment and no indication was given as to when the test might be carried out.

After days of eating hospital food, we enjoyed a veritable feast with Indian wine and Kingfisher beer in the hotel before going to bed. No matter what, we were still celebrating another milestone, that of being discharged. The following day, despite being up four times during the night, we felt rested enough to take on the challenges ahead. The Corion Clinic had emailed us the documents Seán was to collect from them, so that we could check them in advance to ensure everything was included. But again, we spotted a mistake: our documents destined for the Irish embassy had the Canadian embassy's address on them. We phoned the clinic to ensure that the correction would be made by the time Seán arrived there. While he went off, I attended to other more pressing needs like washing underwear and baby clothes, not the easiest of jobs to do in a small hotel room and an even smaller bathroom, but needs must. The best part was that because it was so hot outside they dried in a jiffy hanging out on the open window.

Later in the day when there was still no word from the embassy about the DNA test Seán resorted to phoning them. We had decided Seán would be our point of contact from here on in with the embassy, as I hadn't exactly hit it off with their representative. To be perfectly honest, I found their staff to be condescending and unhelpful to us, and I was still annoyed with the attitude shown to us during the previous calls. Unperturbed by Seán's call, it was clear they were not going to respond to our request to arrange the test as a matter of urgency. She simply said they would revert when arrangements were made. Clearly we didn't matter to them. It didn't matter that we were in a foreign country alone; it didn't matter that we were paying for accommodation in two cities; it didn't matter that our hotel room was too small and uncomfortable for us all to live in; it didn't matter that we couldn't take Donal and Ruby outside for a walk in the fresh air. Our children didn't matter, and we didn't matter.

Because a lot of the affidavits had already been prepared and sent to us in advance of the DNA test, we knew one of them would have to be amended by the solicitor before the test could go ahead. It needed to be dated, and of course as yet we still didn't know what the date was going to be. However in tandem with that, we were acutely aware that we still needed to be prepared in case we got the call to go for the sampling at short notice or maybe at a time when our solicitor was unavailable. To ensure we were ready to go at the drop of a hat, our solicitor offered to amend the date and send on the affidavit to us every morning on a day-to-day basis until we got the call.

We got the call next morning telling us to be at the Clinical Diagnostic Clinic that same day at 3 p.m. for the DNA testing. We knew it would take us about two hours to get to the clinic, so Seán headed to the taxi rank just outside the hotel to do the usual haggling. This was where he met Tiawai. Tiawai was a tall, clean-cut, shaven-headed Hindu taxi driver of around 60 years old. His car was immaculate but as usual the seat belts didn't go around the car seats. However, he drove carefully and competently pointing out landmarks and giving us little snippets of history here and there as we drove towards the clinic. A friendship was quickly forged and from there on in we relied on Tiawai to bring us everywhere. He lived outside the city and left his home every morning at 5 a.m. to take the bus to work as a taxi driver. He told us about the small bit of land he had where he grew his own vegetables. His family were grown up and gone and now it was just himself and his wife at home. Every day he was dressed in well-worn but immaculately clean and neatly pressed clothes. He told us that despite being a Hindu he enjoyed a whiskey every night. Over the ensuing days and weeks, as Seán and Tiawai shared the front seats of the taxi, they chatted about everything and anything, but always the conversation started with, 'You have a drink last night?'

Tiawai knew all the shortcuts in Mumbai and used them wisely as we wound our way towards the upmarket tourist area where the clinic was located. We drove past the Gateway of India and the misplaced opulence of the Taj Mahal Palace Hotel. The area was idyllic with the Arabian Sea glistening to our right and cricketers playing their national game in the large green parks to our left. On down towards the bay and in the distance we could see the one and only Mosque in Mumbai, sitting out on the water accessed only by a long narrow pedestrian pathway. Tiawai explained how this area was always extremely busy, as hundreds of pilgrims made their way to the Mosque every day. We continued on our way through the narrow streets lined with lots of tiny tourist shops, pubs, restaurants and cafes. This area was apparently also very popular for weddings. In India, marriages are fantastically colourful and theatrical displays. When a wedding is held, the music on the streets can be heard long before the wedding procession comes into sight; the beat of the drums gets louder as the marriage procession draws ever closer. The groom, in full ceremonial dress and mounted on a white festively adorned stallion, usually arrives surrounded by throngs of men, women and children. Everyone is dressed lavishly, laughing, singing and dancing to the beat of the music. His bride, dressed in her beautifully colourful and ornate wedding costume, painted with henna and wearing the obligatory gold jewelled bangles, rings and necklaces, waits patiently for him at the ceremonial venue surrounded by her relatives and friends. On arrival, trays upon trays of food are served while the dancing and celebrations go on well into the small hours, proving that the Indians like the Irish certainly know how to party.

At the Clinical Diagnostic Centre, we paid the Rs. 3,000 (€42) as the fee for taking the samples and also a consulate fee of Rs. 3,600 (€50) for the witness to attend the testing. She had not yet arrived but had phoned to confirm she was on her way. It was the same lady that had been led on a wild goose chase by the embassy the week previous. We were ushered promptly into the office where two doctors were waiting to complete the documentation and prepare for the tests. There was a raft of documents and affidavits to be completed and signed before the test would be carried out. I handed over all the passport photos as well as Seán's passport. Neither my passport nor signature would be required for I did not exist.

Shortly after, our witness arrived. She was a broad smiling Indian lady who told us she had visited Ireland several times and loved our country. Swabs for the DNA testing were to be taken from the inside of Donal and Ruby's mouth, and we had been told not to give them any food or drink for a specific number of hours prior to the testing, a difficult task with two small hungry babies. We had fed them at the twelfth hour, hoping they would be pacified long enough for the swabs to be taken. We need not have worried that we had fed them too close to the appointment time because of the delay with our witness arriving and completing the documentation. The issue now was that the lads were beginning to get hungry again and were letting everyone know it.

The swabs were taken promptly. Each one was carefully placed in its container and sealed for storage and transportation together with the relevant documentation. They would be transported to the OQPS initially and from there they would be transported to the UK for the actual testing to be carried out. We could not get our heads around this convoluted process and wondered why there was no clinic in a position to carry out this type of testing in Ireland, instead of having to send the samples to the UK. At every stage of this process there presented more questions than answers. Before we left we gave our witness our address telling her next time she was in Ireland to look us up, and we meant that sincerely.

By the time we got back to the hotel the day was slipping, and it was time for more bottle washing, kettle boiling and formula making. We now had two different types of bottles on the go to ensure we didn't get the different formulas mixed up, but the risk of running out of formula was something we had to be on top of throughout our stay. It was proving to be quite difficult to get the formula locally in the small shops or pharmacies, and there was no large supermarket near the hotel. When we needed to replenish the formula, we usually had to get a taxi to go to any number of pharmacies in the hope that one of them would have what we needed. Some pharmacies had the formula one day but the next time they wouldn't have any, or they might only have one box or one type in stock. It was always very much hit and miss. On one occasion, Seán and Tiawai had to try three different pharmacies before eventually getting one box of formula. It did become a bit easier when we moved to Pune as there were a number of pharmacies and a supermarket close by which generally stocked the various brands.

40

COMMERCE

We were on our way back to the hospital to see Dr Soni in OPD where we hoped she was going to give us the all-clear to head to Pune. All our business at this stage was concluded in Mumbai, and our plan was to travel to Pune the next day to start living just a little bit like normal people instead of out of suitcases.

Taxi and rickshaw journeys in India were still a wonder to us. Each trip was a new adventure, and this one to the hospital was no different. The only time that the traffic in Mumbai ever seemed to slow down or give way was when the sacred cow rambled onto the streets. Every day, cows aimlessly meandered along footpaths and streets oblivious to the chaos they caused the commuters. We were stopped in traffic to let one such beast pass when out of the corner of my eye I spotted movement on the path just beside the car. I did a double take when I saw it was the scurry of rats scrambling around on a rubbish heap just a few yards away. There must have been twenty or more of them running all over the place, paying no heed whatsoever to the people passing by, who, in turn, took no notice of the rats. Every day brought a new readjustment to living in India, but some things I would never be able to readjust to.

Something else we also noticed was that in India there appeared to be a very methodical and organised manner in how markets were set up and operated. Stalls selling the same type of produce were set up side by side; for example, all the fish stalls were located together on one street, the meat stalls on

another, clothes stalls on another and so on. It made absolute
sense, as customers could easily view what was on offer and
more importantly could easily compare prices to ensure they
got a bargain. As we continued on our journey we passed by the
fish market: a long line of vendors selling all manner of fish out
of makeshift stalls at the side of the road. The women, as usual,
sat cross-legged, swatting the flies away. Sometimes they had a
small fire to generate smoke rather than heat. It seemed the
smoke dispelled the flies, which were really a minor annoyance
to the vendor. The next street had stalls selling chickens that
were all hanging by the neck from racks overhead. There were
eggs in trays and what seemed to be skinned rabbits or hare or
indeed maybe something else entirely unfamiliar to us also on
display. Then rounding the corner, long tables came into view.
These were laden down with vegetables and fruit, all manner of
produce in a blaze of colour. Some items we didn't know the
names of let alone how to cook them, but it was an experience
to admire the display.

The smell of spices wafted in the air: cinnamon, star anise,
ginger, green cardamom, the much rarer large black cardamoms
and garam masala. These were the real deal – a mix of specially
selected whole spices carefully measured to create the base for
the fabulous dishes we sampled daily – certainly not to be
confused with the uninteresting powdered variety we get on the
supermarket shelves at home. Curry powder was not something
you could actually buy in India nor was it easy to get ready-
blended spices to use as a base for a curry. Our friend Tom, being
an avid lover of Indian curry, had asked me to bring back some
Indian curry powder, but try as I might It was not to be had.
Instead in India each cook combines and mixes their own blend
of spices to create their own particular base for curry. So in the
end, Tom got the same: a variety of spices and a cook book from
India to help him in his quest to make the perfect vindaloo,
which by the way was not to be seen on an Indian menu either!

We passed through Bandra, an area renowned for its teeming
market stalls selling clothes, handbags and shoes. This was a

popular area for tourists to come and shop, as it was also home to many American and western-influenced shopping malls. We drove across town through what was now familiar territory to us as we returned to the affluent area of Powai. Security checked us and we were on our way first to OPD, then the hospital shop to stock up on formula and then to accounts to pay the final bill before heading back to base.

There was a small queue as we took our seats to wait outside the clinic. Another couple with twins had also just arrived. It was obvious they were as a result of egg donation and most probably surrogacy. Inevitably, we made eye contact as you do when you find someone in similar circumstances, and they told us they were from Denmark. They were having their babies' final check before being discharged.

Ruby was first up to be weighed and measured, then she had her umbilical cleaned and checked and her little chest listened to. Everything was clear and all was documented in her record book. Dr Soni asked us about the feeding, making sure we had no difficulties or issues. Next, everything was repeated with Donal. She was happy for us to travel on to Pune, but before we left she gave us details of a hospital and a doctor in Pune should we run into any medical problems. She also asked us to return to the clinic again for a final check-up before we were due to fly home. She wanted to ensure everything was OK for the journey. We found this reassuring, and we were very happy to comply. Dr Soni was always very brusque and abrupt in her manner, but this we now knew was not intended to be rude.

Following the check-up, I left Seán with the lads while I went upstairs to the accounts department to finalise our bill and to get the no-dues letter we needed for the visa applications. There they confirmed that Shobha had been discharged the previous day. The additional money to be paid amounted to Rs. 159,300 which was €2,250. We received a meticulously itemised copy of the total bill which was seventeen pages long. We could only trust and assume all was in order and correct. After paying, I was given the receipts and the required letter. When I got back to the lobby, Seán was chatting to two Canadian guys living in Sweden. They were a gay couple who had come on the same journey as us, to collect their newborn baby girl conceived through the Rotunda clinic. They had arrived in Mumbai the previous night, unfortunately too late for their baby girl's birth. She had decided to make an early entrance, but they were over the moon. They asked loads of questions and wanted to hear all we had gone through and experienced so far. They were staying in an apartment complex very close to the hospital called, The Lalco Residence. We had checked them out initially but found they were too expensive for us. One of guys worked in the Canadian consulate in Sweden, and while they had been referred to the same solicitor as us, they had opted instead to go it alone. They felt he had enough experience to be able to handle the legal aspects himself without having to hire a solicitor in India. We were somewhat dubious of this, but then maybe the legal system in Sweden towards the issue of surrogacy was not as complex or as absent as ours. We were sorry we didn't get their contact details, as we have often wondered how they got on. It was good to chat, to exchange experiences and trade ideas, because without this contact we knew it could be a very lonely and isolating place to be at times.

Finally having stocked up on formula and other bits from the hospital shop, we headed back out to meet Tiawai for the journey back to the hotel and for what was to be our last evening before leaving for Pune. On the way back we had to feed Ruby and Donal. Feeding them on the go was a regular occurrence at that stage. Once back at the hotel, we took our leave of Tiawai, thanked him for his help and explained to him that we would be back in Mumbai soon and we would meet again. Tiawai had already explained that he couldn't do the trip to Pune with us because he only had a taxi licence for Mumbai. His taxi wouldn't have been big enough for us and all the luggage we had accumulated so far anyway. As we shook hands we knew it was not for the last time.

41

SETTLING IN PUNE

The drive to Pune was as expected: nerve-racking. We couldn't secure the car seats and we had read about this particular stretch of road being notoriously dangerous. Seán sat in the front with his seat pushed back just enough to wedge one of the car seats in place and prevent it from moving, while I once again sat between the two seats with an arm around each to hold them steady. We drove out of Mumbai, winding our way up into the mountains towards the city of Pune once again, only this time we had our new family with us.

We took a pit stop about half way to Pune. Our taxi pulled into a lay-by where there were public toilets, a few stalls selling drinks and snacks and a couple of small shops. Seán went in search of the toilets but quickly returned to advise against using them, so it was a case of holding on until we got to our new home. When we arrived back in Pune, it was easy now to see the contrast with Mumbai. Although it was chaotic, with traffic and people travelling to and fro, there was a more spacious and laid-back feel to this city. It didn't feel as crowded. People weren't openly lying on the footpaths, sleeping everywhere and anywhere, and begging was something that was not as obvious either. It was just after lunchtime and to accommodate our luggage we took the larger service lift up to the twenty-second floor. We were then left to our own devices to settle in, unpack and check out our home for the next three weeks at least.

It was as we remembered, bright and very spacious, something we had really missed within the confines of our hotel room in Mumbai. Many of the apartment blocks were still in various stages of construction. From our balcony, we had an expansive view out over the golf course across to the river where, over the coming weeks, we would witness throngs of people herding their cattle into the dark and murky waters where both man and beast bathed.

On that first night we weren't sure what to do about dinner. We didn't know the area yet and we hadn't sufficient provisions to cook. We knew we could have a dinner cooked for us in the apartment complex for only €3 per person if we ordered before 6 p.m. The downside was we would have to go to the communal dining room to eat. This wasn't so easy for us because we had Donal and Ruby to consider. Carrying them up and down with us didn't seem the most practical thing for us to do. We asked Surendra about takeaway recommendations and immediately he offered to deliver the in-house dinner to us. He was making an exception for us, and it was a kind and thoughtful gesture. However, we also suspected he had an ulterior motive in that he wanted to get a glimpse of our babies. We were right. He doted over them.

Thereafter, we settled into a routine of either ordering food in or we went out to restaurants. Takeaway food was always plentiful, delicious and cheap. The only problem we discovered was that the order had to be placed several hours in advance to be sure it was delivered on time. More often than not and irrespective of how early we ordered, it always arrived frustratingly late. But we were generally preoccupied enough preparing Donal and Ruby for bed or bathing and massaging them. We had learnt that Indian massage was routinely carried out on all babies in India up to the age of three or four, and we had been shown how to do it on Donal and Ruby. In ancient India, Ayurvedic medicine taught the use of infant massage and it is still part of traditional childcare in India. It is a massaging technique carried out daily by mothers and is considered to instil fearlessness, harden bone structure, enhance movement and limb coordination and increase weight. A dough ball made from water and flour is used for the first four weeks until the baby is strong enough to take hand massage. The dough ball is softened each time in almond oil and rolled along the body, paying particular attention to the extremities. So each morning and night we massaged using the routine to bond and get to know every inch of our children.

The lads settled into a routine of waking for two hourly feeds and generally sleeping in between. While the apartment was spotless and cleaners came daily to clean the apartment, make up the bed, change the sheets and leave fresh towels, you couldn't get rid of some pests, in this case the cockroaches. We didn't see them that much by day, but they emerged under cover of darkness, intent on acting like locusts in our kitchen. Anytime we ventured into the kitchen at night and switched on the lights, it was like a dark blanket being torn apart on the ground as they scattered to the four corners. We knew we couldn't eradicate them for they were more a part of the furniture than we were, so we could only manage the problem. We couldn't leave food open or out on the countertop, only sealed containers of basic necessities such as coffee, biscuits and porridge. We only kept sealed milk and beer in the fridge because the pests managed to break in there too. The steriliser had to be sterilised daily, and we had to be vigilant in keeping the lid on at all times. Crockery, cutlery and glasses had to be scalded with boiling water before every use. We stored the formula along with Donal's medicine in sealed containers, and washing our hands about fifty times a day became routine.

Seán and I grew closer than ever as we watched and marvelled in Donal and Ruby growing and developing into their own little personalities. We have a strong belief that Donal and Ruby benefitted enormously from this time of having absolutely nobody else but their parents with them. The bond and love that was nurtured between us during this time was tremendous, as well as developing a routine that we hoped made them feel safe and secure. That's not to say we didn't miss our families, especially Diarmáid, Rián and Tomás. However, if we looked at the positives of that time being away from family and friends then it was that we developed such a strong bond with the lads, a bond that can never be broken. Day by day our confidence in caring for them grew until we were more than capable of caring and looking after both Donal and Ruby on our own for long periods of time. It was around this time that Seán decided he was going to get fit, so before he changed his mind I bought him a pair of shorts and runners to help him get started. Looking down from our balcony on the twenty-second floor, I could pick out Seán very easily in the distance as he jogged around the golf course. Resplendent in the only pair of shorts I could find – bright lime-green coloured – he certainly didn't need the high-vis.

We started to take turns going to the shops for provisions, as we needed lots of bottled water for making up the formula as well as for drinking. There was also always a need for some basic provisions such as nappies, wipes and toiletries. On other days we took it in turns to venture further afield into Pune to one of the shopping malls or to the markets. The taxi would be ordered the evening before and usually cost €6 for a half day or €12 for a full day. The taxi picked us up and dropped us off wherever we wanted to go, then parked up and waited for our return. It worked a treat as we each got to see Pune. One of us would go to a different place each day, and that evening report back to the other about where we had gone and what we had seen. The challenge was for whichever one of us was left with Donal and Ruby for the day, because now they both woke for feeding at the same time and there was only one pair of hands.

One day, it was my turn to explore more of Pune, and I got lost in one of the larger market areas of the city. When the taxi dropped me off I had, as usual, picked a landmark just in case, but as I wandered through streets and alleyways, caught up in the bustling crowds, I lost sight of the landmark and couldn't seem to find my way back. The market seemed never-ending, winding into side streets and alleyways. It was vibrant, noisy and crowded with hawkers selling everything from spices, herbs, incense, smoking pipes, jewellery, pots, pans, clothes, fruit and vegetables. The stalls were so colourful and mesmerising one could easily be forgiven for wandering off and getting lost. The heat was searing and I could feel the sun burning my shoulders and face, despite the sunscreen I had liberally applied earlier. I found myself in some back streets at the edge of the market, amidst barking dogs marking their territory. I wasn't sure if they were wild dogs or not, but I kept my distance and treated them as such. India was full of wild dogs travelling in packs. They were particularly prevalent at night and never afraid of humans. From our apartment we could hear them in the distance, barking and howling every night.

I continued walking and suddenly realised with a jolt I was in the Indian equivalent of Amsterdam's red-light district. Long, narrow, dark streets dotted with small houses and shacks were interspersed with a few meagre shops for good measure. Scantily clad ladies lounged against the open doorways in search of the next business opportunity. Watching and scrutinising me closely as I passed, some bared a toothless smile while others just peered curiously or suspiciously at me. Thankfully no one tried to approach me or bother me. I knew I was completely lost and that I couldn't keep walking aimlessly. I had to try and find the entrance to the market and that meant finding someone who could understand me and hopefully direct me. After asking in vain a few times, I eventually managed to find someone with a smattering of English who helped me find my way back to the entrance where I could get my bearings and find my waiting taxi.

Being female, alone and lost in an Indian city is sobering and a position I would not like to find myself in again. I would have to be more careful. When I recovered, I told Seán where I had ended up. I knew immediately he didn't believe me, for it was hard to believe that with all the religious temples dotted on every street there could be a red-light district smack in the middle. No way! He genuinely thought I was having him on until one day he stumbled upon some public toilets and found himself being propositioned and then it all unfolded before him.

Our washing machine was a luxury and was on the go daily. Drying was an easy task, as everything dried so quickly on the balcony. While we did have air conditioning in the apartment, most days it was pleasant enough just to open the sliding doors and let the warm breeze waft in from the balcony. One particular day I had tons of washing out and while the lads slept I settled back to check emails. Hearing a loud but unfamiliar noise like a plane or helicopter coming closer, I glanced out. I couldn't see anything, so I turned back to the business of emailing. As the noise persisted and seemed to become louder I moved to the balcony to investigate but couldn't see anything in the sky. Suddenly I noticed blackness in the sky over a number of apartment blocks about eight hundred meters away. At the same time there was a strong wind whipping up from behind the same apartment blocks. The wind moved quickly forward enveloping everything in its wake. Rubbish was plucked from the ground and anything else that was loose was sucked up and up into this whirling void.

Somewhere in my head it dawned on me that it was a tornado. I needed to move. It was heading for us, driving forward at speed, crashing into everything and eating all it could. Jesus! I had only ever seen these in films. I only managed to grab some of the clothes before shutting the balcony doors. Inside, the light faded and the wind closed in around us, whipping our clothes and everything else that wasn't nailed down from the balcony, and then it was gone as quickly as it had arrived. Later, and according to Surendra, it was only a mild tornado and nothing to be worried about at all. Apparently they get significantly more severe hurricanes and tornadoes, something I hoped never to witness after that day.

One of the strangest ways we amused ourselves was reading the newspaper. *The Times of India*, one of the most reputable papers in India could be bought for Rs. 3 equivalent to four cent.

We sometimes bought the English version. It wasn't very well translated, but it did give some news on what was happening in the world around us. We soon discovered the best part of the paper was the classifieds. The following are a few examples that amused us greatly:

> Brown Sedan. Not very memorable. Easy to drive through traffic. Rear windshield/tail lights/boot have recently suffered minor damage. Engine number and chassis number have been filed down to reduce weight and increase fuel efficiency. Bring cash in unmarked bills and meet at Old Mill Compound on Sunday, at midnight.

> Battle-scarred police jeep. Front grill and bonnet have 45' diameter holes cut into it in unique pattern. Reason for selling: minor damage suffered during high-speed chase in the course of duty. Free wireless radio and siren. For enquiries please dial 911.

> Top-of-the-line luxury car. Bangalore registration. Car guarantees entry to almost all popular nightclubs and select cricket grounds. Has been the subject of many successful paparazzi hunts. Comes fitted with minibar, LED TV, gaming console and jacuzzi. Suspension might need to be replaced. Buyers please mail me. To see car, Google 'prince of better times' or #princeofbettertimescar on Instagram.

My favourites were these two:

> URGENT. Super-luxury SUV for immediate sale. Lucky number. Fancy colour. Windows tinted 'Impenetrable Black'. Back seat is spacious enough for quick auditions of upcoming starlets. Looks new, apart from the minor skull-shaped dent on front bumper. Price no bar. Call me on XXX or mail whatwasIthinking@buymysuv.com.

2012 model sporty car. Has lots of things added on the side, back and front. Dangerously fast. Very loud when started. Price no object. Car must not be home when son returns. Happy to sell as individual parts too. Call XXX URGENTLY.

They were priceless and clearly showed us that the Indian people have a quick and sharp wit comparable to our own.

42

LEGAL WRANGLING

Our solicitor planned on using the same templates already prepared and used for the Irish person who had gone through the process in India just before us. As such, we expected no surprises with our application for the emergency travel documents. We reviewed the Irish Guidelines again to ensure we had included everything, and we checked the documentation from the clinic and hospital as well as the affidavits required. Seán, as the biological parent, had to sign a declaration stating that on return, he would (a) report to the HSE and (b) issue court proceedings in Ireland. The latter would be to ratify his legal status in relation to guardianship of Donal and Ruby.

Our final job was to complete the passport application forms for Donal and Ruby, which had to be notarised or witnessed. The consulate arranged for these forms to be couriered to us, and we completed the forms in line with the instructions enclosed. Now we had everything we needed, including the affidavits signed by Shobha and her husband. Everything was ready to be submitted to the Irish embassy for processing and forwarding to the Irish passport office.

The file didn't go anywhere but was returned to us. The embassy had a problem with the affidavit from the doctor who took the DNA sampling. The Irish Guidelines required that the doctor taking the DNA samples must complete an affidavit stating:

- Their name.
- Their profession.
- How they were satisfied as to the identity of the person/s giving samples.
- Confirming that the samples were placed in secure containers.
- Confirming that the samples were transferred directly to the laboratory.
- Stating that the samples were not given to the persons being sampled.
- Stating by what means the samples were forwarded to the laboratory.

Each of these specific questions had to be addressed separately in the affidavit. Our solicitor made the mistake of omitting one of the questions, and we made the mistake of not picking up on it. It meant the affidavit had to be drawn up again and couriered to the Diagnostic Clinic for completion again by the doctor. On hindsight, the only way to ensure there were no errors was to take every specific question and requirement contained in the Irish Guidelines and insert them absolutely word for word, verbatim into the affidavits. Redone, we again submitted the file to the embassy, now satisfied that everything was correct and all required documents were included. They forwarded the file to the passport office in Dublin for processing.

The file was returned again. This time the embassy called to say the Irish passport office would not accept the passport applications because both Seán and I completed Section 7 pertaining to parents. However, as I am not recognised as a parent of Donal and Ruby, I should not have completed or signed the forms. Only Seán as the biological father had an entitlement to sign any document on behalf of Donal and Ruby. Neither the embassy nor consulate had provided any specific instructions for their completion, so we had just gone ahead and completed them as per the instructions on the forms. The solicitor could not have foreseen this issue, as the person who went before us was single and this issue had not arisen. However, we felt the Irish embassy should have picked up on this when reviewing our file. Instead they considered it satisfactory and processed it as such.

Another set of forms were couriered to us and this time only Seán signed them. Again the embassy processed the file to the passport office in Dublin, and we waited. Again the file was returned to us with yet another issue. It seemed the goalposts had changed in a few short months and now what the Irish Guidelines stated was no longer acceptable:

> Where the surrogate mother is not a fluent English speaker, it will be necessary for her to sign both the application form and a certified translation, or provide an affidavit in her own language stating that she consents to an Irish travel document for the child being issued to the commissioning father.

We had provided this affidavit as well as an affidavit from our solicitor stating she had translated all documentation to Shobha and her husband in their language, Hindi. However, while this had been previously acceptable, it was not any longer. Now the passport office wanted every piece of documentation and affidavit to be translated into Hindi, served to and signed by Shobha and her husband before we could proceed. They hadn't mentioned this when they raised the issue about the passport application forms, and now it would seem they didn't trust our solicitor to have completed and signed an affidavit confirming she had translated all documentation to Shobha.

The Irish embassy was obviously unaware of this new change to the requirements, as they had been satisfied to process our file to the passport office. So why were they not informed of this change? This was the third time our file was returned. Even though we tried to argue this particular issue was not stated in the Irish Guidelines, it was to no avail. We had to go back and get our solicitor to draw up all of the documentation and affidavits again but this time translating them all into Hindi and serve them on Shobha and her husband. Because Shobha had already been discharged from hospital and was now at home, we had to go back to Dr Kadam and ask her to arrange for Shobha and her husband to return to the clinic to be served the papers. All in all this change set us back significantly, costing us another eight days. For the fourth time our file was again submitted and we crossed our fingers. This time it was good news when the embassy emailed to say the emergency travel certificates for Donal and Ruby were sanctioned. Seán set out at 5 a.m. to travel to the Irish consulate in Mumbai to collect them and pay the applicable fee of Rs. 2,200 (€30). As well as the emergency travel documents, the embassy also issued us with a letter to be given to the Foreign Regional Registration Offices (FRRO) stating that they supported our application for exit visas for Donal and Ruby. We had to agree that once we had the visas and we were ready to depart, we would inform the embassy of our travel arrangements, specifically our flight details so that they could inform the HSE and any other relevant Irish authorities of our impending arrival in Ireland with our two babies. Before we had departed India the Irish authorities knew we were on our way.

We were now ready to apply to the FRRO for the exit visas for Donal and Ruby. We knew that exit visas could be issued in a day or two, but we also knew we might run into difficulties because the following week was Diwali, the festival of lights. This is one of the largest and brightest Hindu festivals of the year, even bigger than our Christmas and New Year put together, and everything is closed down for the duration, over a week. We had an extremely tight time frame. If we didn't get the exit visas over the course of a couple of days we were facing another long delay of up to a week. But to even get into FRRO we first had to make an appointment online. Our solicitor booked the next available appointment which was Monday, 28 October at 10 a.m. In the meantime, we still needed to gather up some additional documents for FRRO namely:

- Our marriage certificate or a declaration as evidence of our marital status.
- The online application form for the FRRO appointment.
- The original receipt, and not a scanned copy, for all of the documents submitted to the Irish embassy.
- Evidence that we were residing at an address in Mumbai.

The declaration of marital status had become a recent requirement as part of the new Indian Visa Guidelines. It did not matter that we had commenced the surrogacy process prior to this becoming a requirement; once the guidelines were implemented we had to comply. While we were not married we had a letter from our solicitor in Ireland supporting our common-law husband and wife status, and we had a letter from the clinic stating we were what they called a 'live-in' couple, again supporting our status as a couple in every sense. The clinic had also given us a letter stating that they had submitted our names to the FRRO as having commenced the surrogacy process prior to the Indian Visa Guidelines being implemented, and as such should be regarded as exempt from having to comply retrospectively. However, the clinic stressed to us not to give over this letter to the FRRO unless asked specifically for it. We were unsure why this was, but presumably because the clinic could be taken to task on this.

Our solicitor agreed to make several copies of everything for us and once back in Mumbai would courier them to our hotel, along with a printout of our online appointment with the FRRO. We made sure to take four copies of everything with us going to the FRRO as well as a full set for taking home. We only had five days to go before we were due to fly home.

At this point we needed to add Ruby and Donal to our flight tickets. I couldn't seem to complete the process online, so I ended up phoning British Airways. They were very accommodating in making the changes which cost only about €100. They also recommended booking the bassinettes for the lads, as they only had so many on each flight. With that done, I phoned Aer Lingus to add the lads to that leg of the journey. We knew we were probably taking a chance making these changes when we still didn't have the exit visas, but if we left it to the last minute, we were afraid we wouldn't get the lads on the flight and we'd end up being delayed further. All we could do was keep the fingers crossed that there would be no more delays and we'd make our flight.

Our plan now was to travel back to Mumbai on Sunday, 27 October and go to the FRRO the next morning to apply for the exit visas. We envisaged our application taking two to four days, and then we would be on the flight home as planned on Friday, 1 November. We were also acutely aware that things could still go wrong. We knew all too well how slowly things progressed in India. If necessary, we were ready to pay *chai-pani* (a bribe) to get things processed quicker. We had been told on numerous occasions that bribery was never accepted in India. However, it seemed that if you worded your sentences carefully while offering *chai-pani* it would be accepted, though not as a 'bribe' per se. It would also never be acknowledged as having occurred.

The last part of our stay in Mumbai was going to be short, so we decided to treat ourselves and booked into the four-star Sea Princess Hotel, directly across from the Emerald Hotel. We had eaten there one evening and knew it was a lot more spacious and comfortable than the Emerald. There was also a pool and lots of secure outdoor areas to walk and relax in. It was more expensive certainly, but we felt it was worth it just for the chance to wander outside in the fresh air with the lads, and anyway it was only for a few days.

A few weeks earlier, we had arrived in India with two suitcases and some hand luggage. Now we had ten pieces of luggage! Seán Malone had even bought swings for the lads, the kind that you hang from an overhead beam. I kid you not! He said they were two for one and a steal at the price. He just couldn't leave a bargain behind.

43

RETURNING TO MUMBAI

Arriving back in Mumbai that Sunday, we were again greeted by people who could smile against a backdrop of hustle and bustle, chaotic traffic and toxic fumes of pollution. Half-clad, downtrodden people begged amidst a myriad of colour, smells and noise that assailed and overpowered the senses. At the Sea Princess, our first impressions were positive as we were presented with floral garlands placed around our necks and offered a drink of cool sweet coconut milk. Rahoul, the front-of-house manager, checked us in and arranged for some of our luggage to be stored in the basement while the rest was brought to our room.

As we checked in we remembered to ask for the letter showing proof of our address in Mumbai to complete the file for the FRRO. We paid for the hotel in advance, and the receipt was given to us as proof of our address. Once up in the room, we discovered that there was no cot and none were available. We had requested one when booking the room but unfortunately they had already been allocated. None would be available for another two days.

However, the hotel staff prepared a makeshift cot, which by the time they were finished was akin to Colditz Castle; no baby was going to escape. It was raised to our bed level and completely encased with homemade bolsters made out of rolled up blankets and sheets. They were going all out to ensure our babies were protected. Maybe they were adept at this, but either way they had clearly gone to a lot of trouble for us.

The room was not large, but it was much more spacious than the Emerald, certainly more than sufficient for our short stay. It boasted the usual facilities, and complimentary bottled water was provided and replenished several times a day. The hotel staff were courteous and friendly. More importantly, they responded to our every need promptly and expertly, and we were to have many over the coming days. Each morning, when we arrived for breakfast accompanied by the lads in the double buggy, staff immediately cleared a path for us and found us a table, irrespective of how busy the dining room was. Similarly, they helped with shopping, organising taxis, lifting the buggy up and down steps and even rushing ahead of us to have the elevator doors open and waiting for us. They made our stay so much more pleasant. The large open foyer with lots of comfortable seating offered a pleasant alternative place to sit in the evenings. Outside, we enjoyed many a drink in the evenings while watching the spectacular sunsets over the Arabian Sea. We were spoiled with all the outside space available to stroll with the buggy. There was private access to the beach from the back of the hotel. The gate was locked and manned by security staff letting hotel guests in while keeping locals out. The beach front was long, sandy and very inviting, but looks can be deceiving. We were advised not to swim, paddle or walk barefooted in the sand because of the high level of pollution. On our first trip in January, we had ventured onto the beach for a walk and were shocked to see men urinating openly, rubbish strewn around and dogs defecating everywhere. This time we admired from a distance.

The sea reminded us of home and our beaches, the White Strand and Spanish Point. Unlike our wild Atlantic Ocean, the Arabian Sea seemed to be forever tranquil, shimmering under the searing heat of the sun. We longed for home. The hotel was on a flight path and every ten minutes we could see planes flying low, some displaying the British Airways logo. Without a word spoken, we'd glance at each other, knowing instinctively what the other was thinking: someday soon, very soon, we would be up there too homeward bound. The locals strolled up and down the beach every day looking in over the high wall. Some stood and stared probably envious of the guests relaxing and having drinks by the pool, while others wandered back and forth glancing over and waving. They must surely have been wondering about this other side of life, a world which would forever elude them.

Directly across the main drag from the hotel, amidst some very expensive modern shops, was a colony: an Indian term for a small local community. Apparently there are millions of these colonies all over the cities of India: places where people live, work, do business and socialise. This particular colony was located down a long narrow street off the main Juhu Tara Road, and there people lived in small huts, shacks or stone houses. They operated their businesses from the front of their huts and stalls, selling everything from fish, eggs and chickens, tobacco, bric-a-brac, toys, fruit and vegetables. Small businesses such as the tailor, the barber shop and the tea houses all vied for customers. Cattle, donkeys, cats, goats and dogs roamed the narrow streets while small children ran and played amongst them. Older children and teenagers sometimes wandered out onto the main thoroughfare to sell everything from second-hand books to make-up, perfume and clothes; all were excellent quality knock-offs at a fraction of the price.

The atmosphere in the colony was similar to that of a busy bustling market. Seán and I had gone there on a number of occasions, but we ventured separately as you couldn't actually wheel a buggy anywhere in Mumbai. Footpaths were generally hazardous with broken uneven areas, gaping holes, garbage and rats rummaging around. Once, Seán passed a huge pile of discarded and rotting vegetables at the entrance to the colony. He saw two donkeys scavenging through the mass of rotting food, and a few feet further on he came upon a frail elderly man in rags down on his hunkers picking and eating from the same decaying mass. He caught this on the camcorder and when he showed it to me, the sight of this man and beasts competing for food, for life, while daily life carried on heedlessly around them, penetrated deep into the soul.

Seán visited the taxi rank hoping to meet Tiawai again. Taxi ranks in India are vastly different to those in Ireland where the drivers queue in an orderly fashion. Here taxis park up in no particular order. As they wait for a fare, they abandon their vehicles and gather around a makeshift table and some benches playing cards, smoking, dozing comfortably and whiling away the time. Nearby, there is the mandatory stall selling traditional tobacco wrapped inside a betel leaf. This is bought predominantly by the male population who place it into the side of the mouth, chew profusely to create large amounts of a thick brown liquid and spit gallantly from the windows while driving. It is not a particularly pleasant sight and is even more appalling when sitting in the open backseat of the rickshaw. There always seemed to be serious competition between the drivers to see who could hawk up the largest and brownest spit, and my cringing shock made them roar in raucous laughter and try even harder next time.

As Seán approached, Tiawai stood to greet him, his extended hand accompanied by a nod and broad smile. Seán explained that we had our twins with us, outlined our plan over the coming days and booked him to bring us to FRRO the following morning. Donal and Ruby would be travelling with us, as FRRO needed to check their identity against their emergency travel documents. Tiawai was not like other taxi drivers; he was always on time for us. We'd like to think this was because we had developed a friendship with him over time. We had told him what we were doing in India from the start, and he knew the importance of us getting our documentation sorted as quickly as possible. He also knew we relied upon him to get us from A to B as quickly and as safely as possible. We paid him well for that service, but it was the respect we showed him and the trust we placed in him that seemed to matter more.

44

FOREIGN REGIONAL REGISTRATION OFFICES

Our appointment for the FRRO was at 10 a.m. We wanted to be early despite knowing that the appointment time was completely irrelevant anyway. While we hoped the wait wouldn't be too long, especially as we had Ruby and Donal with us, we had still packed enough baby supplies to last a two-week holiday. Fully expecting an all-day wait, we had also packed plenty of bottled water and reading materials for ourselves.

We were acutely aware this was the stage of the process where we were most likely to be reprimanded for travelling to India on a tourist visa. We aimed to argue this issue on the basis that we had already entered into the surrogacy process before this requirement became mandatory. However, we also knew our arguments would probably be futile. We didn't know how we would be reprimanded or penalised; we just hoped it would not end up delaying us any further in India.

We had also been forewarned about a particular official in the FRRO who apparently was difficult to deal with and who operated a no-tolerance policy. Of all the staff in the department, he was the person we didn't want to meet. In fact, he had only recently returned from suspension following an investigation into allegations he made against a man whom he had accused of child trafficking. When these allegations were made initially, they had resulted in the man being jailed pending an investigation, the outcome of which proved that the allegations were without foundation. On the one hand, we were appalled to hear this story and obviously apprehensive, but on the other hand, there was a sense that this man was at least vigilant and aware of the potential for abuse and trafficking. Given our own country's appalling history of child abuse, we were acutely aware that surrogacy could be used for the gratification of abusers, therefore all the more reason for strict controls within the FRRO and for legislation and regulation in our own country. It would appear that while the accusations made by the official were unfounded he had made them in good faith, but then one had to presume that the fact he was suspended might deter other officials from acting on or reporting their suspicions. Despite all this, we still hoped against hope we didn't get this official to deal with our case.

We were shocked to find the area around the FRRO building completely congested with hordes of people converging on these government offices. Apparently there were a variety of departments within this government building dealing with all manner of public issues. We exited the taxi and navigated surprisingly quickly to the front door, as people automatically stepped aside when they saw our cargo. We were required to sign in and a lift took us to the third floor where the FRRO office was located. Seán took up position in the queue to check in while I sat in the large but very crowded waiting room. A staff member leafed through our file, briefly checking that each required document was present and then passed the file to a senior official to process while we waited our turn. There was no air conditioning, and while the windows were open throughout the building, they served no respite to the humidity and stifling heat in the room. There was no priority given to the elderly or those with children. We just had to sit it out. We watched people coming and going, ordinary people like ourselves, all in the same situation, all seeking exit visas. We soon got talking to a family from Australia and a couple from Singapore. The Singaporean couple had their baby through the Corion Clinic two weeks previously. They were being issued with their exit visas that day. Their daughter was only fourteen days old and already they were on their way home, while here we were still struggling almost seven weeks later.

A young women travelling with the Aussie family approached us and asked what clinic we had used. Talk about an opening line, we were really that obvious? She was a sister of the intended mother and was certainly well informed about surrogacy. She asked us lots of questions and told us about their own situation. The couple and their extended family had just arrived in Mumbai and were at the FRRO to register their arrival. They also had another daughter with them born through surrogacy three years previously, who was full of health, youthfulness and energy. At that time they had four pre-embryos transferred and became pregnant with twins, but sadly they lost a baby boy at birth. They had used their remaining frozen pre-embryos and this time around they were expecting another baby in just a few days' time. In that moment in the waiting room, it was amazing to see four children and another on the way, all conceived through surrogacy.

Three hours later, Seán's name was finally called. He followed the officer down a corridor while I waited outside with Donal and Ruby. It was like they knew the score they were so good, taking their bottle in turn, burping and sleeping. There was nowhere to change a nappy so I just did it in a corner of the room as best I could. For a government department that dealt consistently with parents and babies, it was significantly lacking in facilities.

Seán asked if I wanted to hear the bad news or the bad news. We had been allocated the dreaded official, and while there was no mention of the tourist visa, the receipt from the hotel, presented as proof of an address in Mumbai, was not sufficient. Instead of a receipt we needed a letter from the hotel specifically stating and confirming that we were residing in the hotel, and it had to be on headed notepaper. We phoned the hotel to ask them to either fax or email through the letter required, but it was now lunchtime and there was no one available in the hotel office to do this. So we waited through lunch and another forty-five minutes before phoning the hotel again. This time we were assured the letter would be written and faxed over to the FRRO. We waited, checking every so often, but still nothing arrived. Over an hour later, we again phoned the hotel. They hadn't realised the urgency of our request and thought it was something that could be done later in the afternoon. As Seán was animatedly impressing upon them the urgency of getting the letter sent immediately, the dreaded official dealing with our case appeared to tell us he was finished work for the day and we would have to return tomorrow to continue the application process. It didn't matter now if the letter arrived or not, we could do nothing more for that day.

On the way back to the hotel we explained to the ever-patient Tiawai what had happened and tried to figure out the best strategy for the next day. We didn't want to take Donal and Ruby back to the FRRO to sit around for another full day, so we decided that Seán would go first thing on his own the following morning. I would be on standby at the hotel with the lads ready to travel to the FRRO if things progressed. Tiawai arranged for a taxi friend to be available to pick us up at short notice. Back at the hotel, Rahoul was waiting to apologise about the mix up with the letter and also to hear how we had got on at FRRO. We explained we had to return again and the importance of having everything in order for the FRRO, including the letter from the hotel. Rahoul made it his business to personally organise the letter for us. He gave us his business card so that we could make direct contact with him if we needed anything else. From that day on, every time we arrived back to the hotel, Rahoul was waiting to ask about our progress and to check if he could do anything more for us. We greatly appreciated his help and concern for us.

45

VISA ISSUES

Off again the following morning, Seán and Tiawai planned to be at the offices before they even opened. We were getting anxious now as we edged ever closer to Friday, when we were supposed to be going home, but we weren't at panic stage yet. Diwali, 'the festival of lights', was fast approaching. If we didn't have the visas by Thursday, chances were we would not get them in time for our flights. On a positive note, we felt that once the letter from the hotel was sorted, we would be OK. They hadn't raised any other issue with our application the previous day.

The call came at 11.30 a.m. Everything was going to plan, so Yadav, Tiawai's taxi friend, would be collecting us to go to the FRRO. We hoped to get there before the offices closed for lunch at 1 p.m. because they would continue to process the application until completion. If we were late and the office was closed, it would mean having to wait around outside until they reopened again at 2 p.m. We didn't know if that would leave enough time to complete it that day. Tiawai had already spoken to Yadav and explained the urgency in getting us to the FRRO before lunchtime. He was older than Tiawai and drove with confidence and expertise. He navigated the congested streets taking numerous shortcuts down side streets and alleyways, some barely wide enough to contain the car. He would have given any rally driver a run for their money as he twisted and turned the car, but not at a speed that would be considered reckless or dangerous. As we travelled down through side streets, he nonchalantly pointed out landmarks and places of interest while still managing to maintain his concentration and intent.

Just over an hour and fifteen minutes later we turned onto the side street which housed the FRRO and waiting for us at the top of the road was our friend Tiawai. Unsurprisingly, the street was completely blocked with traffic. There was no way forward, no way back and no place to park. We were at a standstill. The offices were at the top of the road, about five hundred meters away, and it was almost 12.50 p.m. Despondent, I sank back in the seat knowing we weren't going to make it. The back door of the taxi was suddenly yanked open. Tiawai reached in, grabbed Donal's car seat and shouted at me to follow him. It took me only a few seconds to cop on to what was going on, and I followed clutching Ruby's seat to my side and the bag of baby supplies thrown over my shoulder. Boy, was I sorry I had packed so bloody much now! Yadav just stood beside his taxi in the middle of the road gaping after us helplessly. What a sight we must have been: Tiawai and I running like lunatics, tearing down the street, weaving in between cars with two babies swinging off us in blistering heat. Seán was waiting just inside the building, afraid if he came out the doors would be closed. It was like a relay race as he grabbed Donal from Tiawai and ushered us into the lift to the second floor. We had made it. But as we ascended he told me of our next problem.

This time it was the tourist visa. They would process our application and complete the identification process for Donal and Ruby, but they would not issue us with exit visas until they had spoken with the Irish embassy on the matter, and they still wanted us to comply with the criteria for a medical visa. As well as having the letter confirming our status as a cohabiting couple from our solicitor in Ireland, they now required another letter from the Irish embassy confirming that we were married. They also wanted a statement from the embassy confirming that Donal and Ruby were born through surrogacy. Most of the documents submitted, such as the contract and the letter from the Corion Clinic, already proved surrogacy, but still they insisted on another letter from the embassy. It wouldn't be a problem to get that particular letter, but we were worried about their request for a statement of marriage. If we got these letters to FRRO that day then they would issue the visas to us the following morning.

No amount of explaining to the officials that we had already entered the process of surrogacy before the Indian Visa Guidelines were enacted would appease them. The letter from our solicitor stating we were a couple in every sense of the definition was insufficient; we had to be married. We showed them the letter from Dr Kadam submitted to the Indian Department of Health back in July 2013 outlining that we had already commenced the surrogacy programme and as such should be exempt from having to get a medical visa, but they didn't want to know. As far as they were concerned we knowingly entered India on an incorrect visa and in order to proceed any further we needed to comply with the criteria for a medical visa. Ironically, the one criterion we had been most worried about, the need for Ireland to recognise surrogacy in law, was never mentioned. Before we could contact the embassy about these additional requirements, we first had to complete the application and identification process otherwise we would all have to return again the following day. It was getting way too close for comfort now.

This time we waited outside in the hallway, which was not as crowded or as hot as the waiting room. Sitting beside us was a man who seemed decidedly anxious and quite agitated. He was a business man. He had been in India working and was now preparing to go home. Shortly before he entered India, the government had introduced additional legal requirements, one of which was that all foreigners arriving in India on certain types of visas had to register at the FRRO within fourteen days of arrival. This man had not registered so was facing either financial penalties or a denial of an exit visa. Unaware of the change in law, he couldn't get an exit visa and was going to miss his flight home. The company he worked for were trying to resolve the issue but for now he had no option but to cancel his flight and return to his hotel to wait.

We also met an American man of Scottish descent who was living in Goa for the last eight years. He had been married in the USA, but when his wife died he had moved to Goa. He had arrived at the airport the previous evening to fly to Scotland to meet up with his family but was prevented from boarding his flight. Officials told him he did not have the required visa to exit the country. Earlier in the year and while living in India, he had become ill and had heart surgery. Officials now stated that as he was not an Indian citizen and had received medical treatment in India, he needed a medical visa to travel. They would not be deterred from their erroneous belief that he was in India for medical treatment as opposed to residing there. He had been taken to a holding room at the airport and shown CCTV footage of others being detained for similar reasons. Officials instructed him to look at all the sad faces of people prevented from leaving India. He had missed his flight and spent the night in a nearby hotel. He was now trying to sort things out at the FRRO, but it wasn't looking too good for him. Although anxious and concerned, he felt he had an ace card he could play if all else failed; he had a friend who worked in the Indian government who would travel to FRRO to help him.

These brief conversations left us more concerned than ever. Would we be prevented from leaving? Was the shit going to hit the fan now? Seán tried phoning the embassy a few times but couldn't get through, so he left some voicemail messages asking for an urgent call back. We needed to make contact with them and get things sorted before everything closed down for Diwali. If we didn't get it sorted that day or the next, we'd never get sorted before Friday. The official beckoned to Seán to bring Donal and Ruby in for identification where they were duly photographed and formally certified as being Ruby Darina Malone and Donal Fintan Malone. He told Seán we would have to pay a fine of €30 for using a tourist visa, and he stamped our passports to prove we were guilty of this offence. The stamp on our passports could be an issue if we were ever returning to India. We intended to return someday, but not until Donal and Ruby were old enough to understand where they had come from, and by that time our passports would have been renewed. The worst part of the penalty was not knowing whether we were going to get the exit visas on time or not. The FRRO said they would first speak with the Irish embassy on the matter and then would contact us when our visas were ready for collection. All we had now was a tiny sliver of hope that they might be able to contact the embassy that afternoon, and the visas could still be issued tomorrow or Thursday, still in time for our flight. Deflated and disappointed, we returned to the hotel. This was the lowest point of our time in India. We had been hopeful up to that point and certainly had never considered the possibility, until now, that we might not be going home.

The following day, we still hadn't been able to contact the embassy by phone and had received no call back, so we sent an email outlining what was required. We attached our solicitor's letter which explained Section 172 of the Civil Partnership Act pertaining to our marital status in Ireland. In other words, we were trying to convey that as cohabitants we should satisfy the meaning of marriage, and we hoped this was sufficient for the embassy to issue a letter confirming our marital status within the state of Ireland and in accordance with Irish law. We also attached the letter from Dr Kadam regarding our assertion that we should be exempt from being assessed under the new Indian Visa Guidelines.

It took sending the email for the embassy to return Seán's call. They had not received any call from the FRRO, but maybe like us the FRRO call went unanswered. Instead of providing us with any form of reassurance, she was quick to highlight our crime again to us. Once again we explained why we had no option but to apply for the tourist visa, and she then admitted that we would have got the medical visa if we had applied. So why were we not told this when we emailed the embassy in

June? Why was this was not made known to people in advance of applying for visas? Our protestations fell on deaf ears. The embassy accepted no responsibility for their actions or inactions on this matter. She confirmed what our Indian solicitor had told us: there was an agreement in place between the Irish and Indian authorities to issue medical visas to Irish citizens for the purpose of surrogacy. This information was no good to us retrospectively, as she went on to emphasise to us that the FRRO could choose to withhold our visas for anything up to six months. It couldn't get any worse for us. There was no consolation. We had no one to turn to. Alone and unsupported, the phone was put down on us. Dinner that evening was a subdued affair. Both of us were distracted and quietly lost in our thoughts. Neither of us said anything, but we both knew in our hearts we weren't going home on Friday.

46

GOING NOWHERE FAST

All day Thursday we continued to try to make contact with the embassy and the FRRO, but there was no response. We figured the offices were probably closed for Diwali, but we didn't give up. On Friday, the day we should have been going home, we were still making calls in a last ditch attempt. Rahoul knew we were still waiting for the visas, and he kindly arranged a late checkout for us. He reluctantly made us aware that the majority of offices had already closed for Diwali the previous evening. As he saw the stress etched on our faces, he hastily added that a few government departments might remain open that day with limited staff working. We were all packed and ready for the airport as Seán continued phoning for the hundredth time, but as expected there was no answer. On a wing and a prayer, he chanced phoning the consulate in Mumbai, not really knowing what they could do for us. Lo and behold he got through. Urgently, he explained what was required for the FRRO: the letter confirming our marital status and the letter stating Donal and Ruby were born through surrogacy. There was no hesitation. They would issue both letters to the FRRO immediately. Our elation was short-lived, as they reiterated we should be prepared to remain in India until offices reopened after Diwali. We knew it was now time to rebook the hotel and change our flights.

Our family and friends were disappointed about our delay but rallied to help keep our spirits up. We were also in frequent contact with Denise, and we delivered this latest update. She felt that if we were going to be delayed in India any longer than another week, they would return to India to film. We all believed it was crucial to the documentary to let people see first-hand the legal difficulties we were experiencing.

Offices were not due to reopen until the following Wednesday, so this meant a minimum stay of another week which we hadn't budgeted nor planned for. We had to decide whether to stay at the Sea Princess or move across the road to the cheaper option of the Emerald Hotel. If we were to stay at the Sea Princess, Seán would have to use every ounce of his bargaining prowess to secure a good deal. While he went off to meet Rahoul, I started changing our flights. The following week was considered high season, so we had to pay additional charges. All in all, including our Aer Lingus flight changes, we paid more than €2,500 in additional costs, and that was with Donal and Ruby travelling for free. As Seán said, 'that would buy a decent bull or a lot of nappies'. As usual, Rahoul came up trumps and gave us as good a deal as he possibly could. We could remain in the same room but at a slightly cheaper rate, and he threw in free Wi-Fi. All we could do now was sit back and try to enjoy the festival of lights that is Diwali.

On Saturday, Ruby was a little out of sorts and a bit cranky. She didn't have a temperature and there was nothing that we could see wrong, but something had her feeling under the weather. As a precaution, we stayed in the hotel that evening instead of going out to a restaurant. It was certainly no hardship, as the food was excellent as always. Before dinner Seán had to head off to get some formula, this time with a taxi driver named Papu. We had met him at the same taxi rank as Tiawai and started using him at night-time when Tiawai was off duty. Papu was a 'cute hoore' as they say in Kerry: smarmy and a bit of a fly-by-night. When Seán explained that we were around for another week, Papu refused to take any fare that evening. We were somewhat dubious about this seemingly generous offer. There were no free lunches in India, especially not with this guy. Papu did not disappoint. The following evening, when we ventured out to a restaurant, we forgot to agree the fare in advance and ended up paying Papu double what it should have been! There was even one occasion when he offered to organise a lady of the night for Seán. He obviously didn't think much of me! It seemed he ran his taxi business as a cover for some of his other more dubious exploits. Seán relayed the story to Tiawai, who was quick to dismiss Papu as someone who was 'not nice and not into good business'.

I couldn't resist buying some of the lovely, bright, colourful materials in the markets. Now that I had the extra time, I could get some clothes made up. There was a tailor's shop across the street from the hotel, but they were closed for the week of Diwali. Disappointed, I strolled into the colony where I had seen a tailor a few times, sitting hunched over a long bench, working away outside his shack. Takhee Baba specialised in ladies tailoring, according to his sign, so I approached and asked if he was closing for Diwali. He said he wouldn't if he had work to do, so we struck a deal. I gave him the material and showed him what I wanted. No problem, he would phone me when he was finished and would deliver the finished products to the hotel. I ended up with fifteen pieces of clothing perfectly made but for a fraction of what I would have paid at home.

One day Seán met a young man on the street who wished him a happy Diwali. He stopped, and they chatted about Diwali and India in general. He was in his mid to late twenties and very vocal in his condemnation of the Indian leaders and their politics. We had seen a lot of coverage in the news about the Indian government glorifying in the fact they had just spent billions sending a rocket into space in search of Mars. When asked on the national airwaves about the mission and the costs involved, the government claimed that their space programme was so successful it saved lives each year through the early detection of earthquakes and other natural disasters. This claim was refuted in many quarters with many stating it was not about developing early-detection systems, but rather it was a race against China to be the first to land on Mars. India was spending billions just to be the first to land on Mars while as much as 80 per cent of its population starved and lived in squalor. This young man also complained about the corruption in his country and how the politicians continued to live beyond their means; familiar strains of 'When Irish Eyes are Smiling' sprang to mind. He continued to talk about India's huge foreign debt while at the same time the volume of black money (hidden money) was substantial. Seán then told him of our story with the FRRO. His response was that just one *chai-pani* would have had us on the plane home. Maybe he was right.

Another evening, while having dinner in the hotel, we came across a group of six men, all friends with very strong north of England accents. They were in Mumbai for six days to celebrate a double fiftieth birthday. Interestingly, they were all of Indian origin, having been born in the Punjab. Their families immigrated to England when they were all about ten years old. Despite having lived for most of their lives in Birmingham, they were fluent in both languages and able to switch at will from Hindi to English. They were friendly people, out for the craic, and for us they were an interesting diversion from all the crap we had been dealing with. On their last evening, after we had said goodbye to them, one of the men knocked on our bedroom door and presented us with an almost full bottle of Canadian Club whiskey, which he hadn't got around to drinking. It was a lovely gesture. Similarly, by the time we were leaving, we hadn't drank much more of it either, so Seán passed it on to Tiawai who we suspect didn't pass it on to anyone else.

One day, while Seán was travelling in a rickshaw to Bandra to buy a few things, he was caught short and needed to pee. But where does one take a leak in Mumbai? There were no public toilets and trying to get into a hotel or any public building with all the security wouldn't work. Eventually he went back to his roots and found a spot between a parked car and a minibus. This reminded him of his annual childhood shopping trips to Limerick with his mother, where the same MO would be deployed.

Moving quickly on, he found an open shop buried at the back of the market in a small shopping mall. The proprietor was playing religious Hindi music and getting ready to celebrate Diwali. He bought enough jeans and T-shirts to last the next five years from this fellow. At the same time, he filmed him talking about Diwali and how he intended to celebrate the festival of lights. This man explained that on Sunday he would be closing his business early, as his wife and family would be joining him at his shop for prayers. Sunday was the most important day of the festival, and after prayers they would all go out to dinner. To conclude the discussion and the sale, he threw in a free T-shirt for Seán. It had a Hindi caption and some specific conditions: apparently while wearing the T-shirt one was forbidden to sin. Seán said he had a mind to send it on to Bertie Ahern, Seanie Fitz or Fingleton, who could wear it without distain or emotion.

The week was spent doing very little. By day we relaxed and swam in the pool. By night we watched the festivities around us, including magical fireworks displays and processions through the streets. There was fantastic music and a carnival-like atmosphere everywhere. One day the beach at the back of the hotel began to fill up with people arriving from early in the morning. They came in their droves with food, tents, ground sheets, kites, candles and lanterns. It was almost like they were setting up home and planning on staying for a while. Fireworks could be seen and heard throughout the day. Live music played from a huge makeshift stage, and street food was sold up and down the beach. All day long and into the night people arrived until there didn't seem to be a square inch of sand left unclaimed. It was another part of the Diwali celebrations whereby everyone gathered on the shore to pray for health and wealth, and then at dawn they would enter the sea to face the sunrise in thankfulness. It was an amazing sight to witness: this mass of people praying fervently while slowly entering the Arabian Sea to behold the rising sun.

As well as sightseeing, discovering parts of Mumbai we had not yet seen, we used the hotel gym and treated ourselves to a few massages in the spa. It was a real treat and only cost Rs. 1,200 (€17) for an hour and a half. According to Seán, the massage he got was 'brutal but brilliant' and he 'could easily do twenty minutes with the Clare team'.

Guests weren't allowed to bring alcohol or food into the hotel. This was presumably to ensure that money was spent solely in the hotel. However, every now and again, we managed to smuggle some beer in for a number of reasons. Firstly, it was far cheaper than buying drink in the hotel bar. Secondly, we didn't particularly want to go to the hotel bar with the lads in tow, and finally, Seán considered a few cold beers an absolute necessity for his sanity. I agreed with him there. I didn't particularly like the beer except for its cooling capabilities, and the wine was far too expensive. One evening, though, I tried a mojito before dinner and was hooked.

47

AFTER DIWALI

The embassy and the FRRO reopened for business on Wednesday, 6 November. News from the embassy that morning confirmed that the documents we had asked for had been sent to the FRRO for processing with our application. Rather than trying to phone, Seán headed down there directly, armed with copies of all the paperwork we had, just in case. We felt the only way to get things moving was to attend in person, that way it might not be so easy to fob him off.

They had the visas ready for collection when Seán arrived, yet they hadn't phoned to tell us. We figured they must have had them ready prior to the holiday period but just didn't give them to us. The consulate had come up trumps with the letters, particularly the letter about our marital status. They just stated in the letter that we were married and didn't bother with the palaver of trying to justify our common-law status. When Seán rang me on his way back to the hotel to say he had the elusive visas, I nearly danced a set round the room I was so elated. I phoned the embassy to confirm our flight details, thanking God we didn't have to change flights again. I began packing, this time for definite. Along with the usual items, I sorted the hand luggage to include a change of clothes in preparation for the Irish weather, a range of baby supplies and our travel and legal documentation. We confirmed with Rahoul that we would definitely be departing on Friday. Our flight wasn't until 2.40 a.m. but Rahoul arranged for us to be able to remain in the room until 4 p.m. He was so good to us.

Thursday, our last full day in India, was spent finalising everything and generally just preparing for home. We checked in online for our flight and printed off our boarding passes, as well as counting and recounting nappies to make sure we didn't run short. We planned on making up the formula before leaving the hotel, just in case we wouldn't be able to get boiled bottled water to use.

Rahoul arranged for the hotel transport to take us to the airport, making sure we would be there well in advance to deal with check-in and immigration. We knew from past experience that getting to the departure gate would be a long and tedious process. As well as checking in our luggage we would have to complete the immigration forms and take our place in the long queue, all that as well as the security checks. We were back at that stage where we were trying to figure out how we were going to manage the luggage as well as two babies, two car seats, a double buggy and a shit load of hand luggage. We would just have to cross each bridge as we got to it. We had checked with British Airways when re-booking our flights, and they said that because our connecting flight in London was with a different airline, we would have to collect our luggage on arrival at Heathrow, get from terminal five to terminal one by train and check in again with Aer Lingus. It was going to be the journey from hell, and for us we felt a physical impossibility. We wouldn't panic; we had crossed worse bridges as It was.

48

ON OUR WAY

Checking out and having our final dinner before leaving for the airport was for us both sad and exciting. We would be sad to leave this country and particularly the wonderful people we had met along the way, but the urge to get home to our families was overpowering. With our luggage loaded, we went in search of the staff to bid them farewell. Many of them had become our friends during our stay. We had said our goodbyes to Tiawai earlier in the day and were surprised to see him dabbing his eyes with a handkerchief as he knelt down before Donal and Ruby. Rahoul and some of the staff waved us off on what was a surprisingly emotional drive through the streets of Mumbai, for what we hoped would not be the last time. Darkness had descended by the time we arrived at the airport, but the heat and humidity was the same. All arrivals and departures are channelled into the airport building through the same gate, and unless you are flying out of the country you are not permitted to enter the terminal building. Before allowing anyone into the building, the security guards check all passports and boarding passes. Hence, there are very long disorganised queues of people trying to get in, as well as those arriving trying to get out. Add to this the hordes of people waiting outside – waving goodbye or vying for the first glimpse of their relative emerging – and you get organised chaos.

The minute we pulled up across from the entrance two young men appeared out of nowhere and started to unload our luggage. They piled it on top of several trolleys they had dragged over with them. We didn't know what was going on and seeing our confusion the driver explained to us, as best he could, that they worked for the airport and would help us get to the correct airline desk. That certainly worked for us for we knew we needed all the help we could get. The young men were obviously well versed in airport etiquette and took the lead, guiding us to the top of the queue and into the building. They did this quite easily by pointing at Donal and Ruby and prompting people to move out of the way to let us through. It was not the first time amidst crowds, confusion and chaos, that people simply moved aside to allow us through without complaint or argument. We were led to the British Airways desk and embarrassingly to the top of the queue. Immediately, a staff member steered us to a desk and began the process of checking us in. Seán then set about trying again to see if we could check our luggage all the way to Shannon. He explained our situation to the steward, who in fairness had reasonable English and could understand us. She agreed to call her manager to talk to us. A friendly and efficient lady, the manager listened patiently to our story and politely said she would see what she could do. At this stage we thought she was just paying lip service to our plight, but she sauntered back to us saying it all was sorted. They would check our luggage all the way through to Shannon. British Airways had come up trumps again. Everything was organised, and we gave the biggest tip of all time to the two men who had helped us. They were still standing, smiling and waving after us as we began to manoeuvre our way towards immigration.

There wasn't any rhyme or reason to the method of queuing. Everywhere was chaotic, with long queues of people presided over by armed security. We filled out the four immigration forms, clutched our exit visas, passports and emergency travel certificates and took our place in line. As we edged slowly forward, a female security guard came striding briskly towards us indicating for us to follow her. We looked at each other, silently wondering if we had done something wrong, and we followed her. She marched brusquely ahead to the top of a queue which according to the sign was for the infirm or disabled; the only other person in the queue was a woman in a wheelchair. We weren't complaining as we were quickly ushered forward to probably the one and only unpleasant looking individual. He glared at us and glowered at her as he told us sternly to get back behind the white line and to come forward individually and only when he beckoned. Retreating with our tail between our legs, we waited while he rummaged, seemingly too busy with paperwork to deal with us.

After punishing us sufficiently for our breach of the white line, he signalled with his index finger as if calling a bold child forward. I went ahead first, pushing the buggy. He then made me reverse again, as he wanted to see Donal and Ruby for identification purposes. When I handed him the documentation he refused to take it, waving his hands about and glowering while telling me to open all the documentation at the relevant pages before handing them to him. He wasn't done there. When completing the immigration form, I had just written our address as the 'Sea Princess Hotel, Mumbai'. However, he wouldn't accept this and insisted on the full address being written on the forms. I went off to one side to complete the forms again, cramming the full address into the tiny space on the forms. When he finally accepted the forms, he then instructed me to take Donal and Ruby's hats off and to wake them up in order to check their identity against their travel certificates. Could he not have as easily checked them without having to wake them up? Maybe he was still reprimanding us for breaching his queue. However overly rigorous he was being, we were certainly not going to question any security measures. The stories we had been told at the FRRO remained fresh in our minds, so we happily did his bidding. He spent a long time scrutinising the penalty stamp imposed on our passports before finally allowing us through. Despite being first in line, it had still taken us forty-five minutes to get through immigration.

Next up was security, located upstairs on the first floor. Arriving at the stairs we were again singled out and ushered down a warren of corridors to a disabled lift. Given the distance we had just walked to get to the lift, it wasn't exactly of much benefit to the incapacitated. It would have been far easier and quicker to just lift the buggy and the luggage up the stairs. Exiting the lift we were met by another member of the airport staff who brought us through the security check. Males were brought to one side and frisked whereas females were frisked in private behind a small curtained cubicle. Seán was finished and through pretty quickly followed by our bags, whereas we took a lot longer. After me it was Donal and Ruby's turn. Their clothes were checked, blankets removed and the buggy was put onto an X-ray machine. It was all very thorough, which was reassuring.

In a matter of ten to fifteen minutes we were on our way to the departure gates. Here we met with more good luck as passengers with children were called forward to board first. The flight was completely full, and unfortunately Seán and I were split up because we were late changing our tickets. There were no seats together where the bassinets were located, and worse still we only had one bassinet, so Donal and Ruby would have to share. We got chatting to the stewards who came forward to help us and discovered coincidentally and unbeknownst to each other that they each had twins: one had 5-year-old twins while her male colleague had 23-year-old twins. The bond this commonality forged between us certainly helped, as they quickly ousted a male solo traveller from his seat so that Seán and I could sit together. Holding Donal and Ruby in our laps in preparation for take-off, we experienced a load of e's: excitement, elation, exhaustion and exuberance.

Denise once asked us when we would raise a glass of champagne and celebrate. Would it be when we conceived or when they were born? Would it be when we got the emergency travel certificates or the exit visas? At the time we said we would celebrate only when we were on the flight home, but now as we were ascending into the night sky looking down at the fading lights of Mumbai, there was no champagne and no big celebration, only a peaceful happiness in our hearts. Tired with the anxiety and toll of the last few weeks, all we yearned for was sleep. We often joke about that flight because it was probably the only flight we ever took together that we did not enjoy a drink or two. The lads normally went to sleep facing each other in their cot, but now they settled head to toe in the too-small bassinet. Before we nodded off, we glanced in to see Ruby with her big toe in Donal's mouth. Both were oblivious to everything around them, happy to be lying close together.

Once in Heathrow and another step closer to home, we set off quickly to catch the train from terminal five to terminal one. We had four hours to kill before our connecting flight, but we didn't know how long it would take us to travel between terminals, and we also needed to change our clothes for our northern climate. We were sitting amongst the vast expanse of high-end, duty-free shops and cafes, in the middle of changing and settling the lads, when we heard a loud American drawl directed towards us. Dressed in canary-yellow trousers and plaid shirt, this short but very rotund American shouted over at Seán, 'Hi, Grandpa. We know one another's story, don't we?' It was one of those moments you couldn't plan if you tried. I nearly fell into the buggy with the laughing when I saw Seán's face, and all I could hear him say was 'let me at him'. He was joking, of course!

The last leg of our journey was Aer Lingus Flight EI381 to Shannon. Shannon Airport is the best airport in the world. Maybe that's something to do with coming home or maybe it's something to do with the informality of a small airport, where everyone is personable and friendly. Whatever it is, there is nowhere else in the world where the guy on passport control would remind you to 'be careful on the roads around Kilmaley for there's a bit of frost'.

There were no bassinets on this leg of the journey due to the short flight time, so we held the lads in our laps for the duration. We didn't mind that and the flight itself was not full so we had the row of seats to ourselves. We were excited about meeting everyone at the airport. We knew Edel was going to be there to film our arrival back on Irish soil. Diarmáid, Rián, Tomás and Marion as well as Donal, Mairéad and David would also be there to greet us. We were relaxing with our own thoughts and finally having that unintentional glass of champagne, complimentary from the staff, but it didn't feel celebratory, it was relief. As the seat-belt sign illuminated to prepare for descent towards Irish soil, right on cue, Donal balked by making a serious deposit, requiring not only a nappy change but a full change of clothes. As the plane continued its descent, Seán managed the situation expertly, impressing all the female stewards on board. Settling back in our seats again and emerging from the clouds, we looked down on our country – our county, our home. It was probably one of the truly emotive and memorable moments in our long and arduous journey, and we savoured every second of it while holding Donal and Ruby in our arms. I believe our real celebratory moment was when the wheels of the plane carrying our family touched Irish soil at Shannon Airport, for at that moment we were home.

49

HOME

Of course it was raining the obligatory rain; that heavy mist that Irish people often refer to as soft rain but would drown you before you knew it. The steps were wheeled to the door of the plane, and below us on the tarmac we could see Edel's camera poised waiting for us. We let the rest of the passengers disembark ahead of us as we struggled to hold the lads and gather our bits and pieces, but once again the staff intervened to take our luggage allowing us to focus on just carrying Donal and Ruby. It was now lashing rain outside. Although the lads were all wrapped up, they were about to experience their first drops of rain. Once down the steps, Seán put Donal's feet gently on the ground before tucking him into the buggy, followed quickly by Ruby. We then turned to hug Edel.

Inside, ground staff were standing by with a trolley to help us retrieve our luggage from the conveyor belt. All we had to do was identify our luggage and they would do the rest. After all fifteen pieces of luggage were loaded, we headed towards passport control. It was such a difference to immigration control in India. As we reached the desk and handed over our passports along with the travel certificates, we were met with a big Irish smile and a 'who have we here' greeting – confirmation that we were really home. We would have liked to keep the travel certificates for Donal and Ruby, but they were a once off and had to be handed over. Leaving behind immigration, our pace quickened as we went through the nothing-to-declare channel towards the arrivals hall. The doors swung open and we could see everyone: a huge crowd of our family and friends who had all travelled and had been waiting so long and so patiently for us were holding banners aloft welcoming us. Seán and Tomás ran towards each other, arms open wide. They had missed each other so much, and it was a magical moment to see them locked together hugging. I was at the same time hugging and kissing Diarmáid and Rlán and introducing them to their new brother and sister. It was such an exhilarating occasion, and it was lovely to see my older boys taking turns to gently and carefully hold Ruby and Donal. It seemed we were there forever hugging, kissing and introducing the lads to everyone. Ruby and Donal cried loudly. Having been used to only Seán and I for so many weeks, they were probably overawed by all the attention. Everything was in hand, Tony and Breda had most of our luggage loaded into their car ready to drop off to us later, while Mairéad and David had reorganised their car to drive us all home.

We chatted endlessly on the drive to Miltown, trying to take in all the news, everything we had missed since leaving for India. It was still raining heavy when we arrived in town just at the unveiling of the Willie Clancy memorial statue on Main Street. It was a humble acknowledgement to a great musician and a moment which would serve to act as a reminder of the day we returned home.

It was hard to settle back as we wandered around the house checking things. Big Donal had the baby cribs assembled for us ready and waiting in our bedroom. We never considered for one moment that Donal and Ruby might not adjust too readily to being separated when it came to bedtime. As we set about unpacking the necessities, we realised in all the fuss at the airport that the holdall with the formula was missing in action. It was now en route with Tony and Breda to Galway. We wouldn't have it back in time, so off Seán went on yet another errand to buy formula, only this time it was to our local supermarket where there would be no problem with supplies. That night, even though we hadn't planned it, Donal and Ruby were on their new formula and we were all ensconced in bed at the very early hour of 8 p.m. We were totally wrecked but Donal and Ruby had other ideas. Having had such an exciting day, discovering they had lots of loving family and friends, and trying to find each other in their separate cribs gave rise to a very unsettled night. They were wide-eyed, bushy-tailed and certainly not ready for sleep. It was the small hours before they finally nodded off, and we followed gratefully. It was their first night of sweet dreams in their own home. The following day the cribs were put aside, and the bigger cot was assembled so that they could both sleep together. At bedtime, we placed them gently at each end of the cot so they wouldn't inadvertently hit or disturb one another. But by morning they had found each other. They had managed, despite being swaddled, to move to the middle of the cot and there they lay together, Ruby with her head on Donal's shoulder.

The next day Seán returned to work while Donal, Ruby and I visited our GP. I had arranged for Mairéad to make an appointment in advance of us arriving home. We didn't think anything was wrong, but I wanted to have the lads checked out to make sure everything was OK. The embassy had informed the HSE of our arrival and they in turn had informed our GP. She told us that the public health nurse would be visiting us at home later that same day. The dust wasn't allowed settle under our feet, and we obviously no longer needed to inform the HSE of our arrival into the country since they were already well aware. The nurses were a brilliant support to us throughout the following weeks and months bringing me right up to speed on everything baby. They gave us lots of books and leaflets, contact phone numbers and encouraged us to call them anytime if we were worried. For us it was reassuring to know they were at the end of a phone if we needed them.

Over the following days and weeks, friends and neighbours called to see Donal and Ruby, all seemingly happy for us. Some scratched their heads in wonderment, convinced we are mad, while others were enthralled. But everyone was completely smitten by our new additions. Every time we went for a walk it took forever, as we were inundated with people genuinely and sincerely wanting to meet us and welcome Donal and Ruby to the town.

50

A CHRISTMAS BOMBSHELL

onal and Ruby's first Christmas was fast approaching and we were really looking forward to spending it quietly at home with our now much expanded family. Of course, despite the fact that Donal and Ruby were too young to understand, we still visited Santa in his grotto and in turn Santa was preparing to visit us at home. Everything was magical.

It was Friday, 20 December when out of the blue I received a call from my work. It was not good news. Despite having been sanctioned with paid leave, the organisation had now decided they were no longer going to continue the paid leave. Not only were they revoking this decision, but they were also going to be seeking to recoup the salary already paid to me since I commenced leave. In essence, this decision meant I would have to return to work immediately. Stunned into silence, I couldn't believe that they could do this, that they would do this, and just days before Christmas, too. It seemed it had suddenly been realised that an error had been made granting me leave. The lack of legislation in Ireland meant they had no obligation to grant me leave, and so on that basis they were reversing their decision.

Putting the phone down, I wondered how an organisation that promoted high standards of care and that spoke of valuing people, putting people first, promoting the rights of people and advocating for the protection of people could treat an employee or indeed anyone in such a way. I always considered myself to be a strong person, particularly having come through some tough life events, but this now reduced me to tears. I wondered how I would cope going back to work while Donal and Ruby were still so tiny and so vulnerable. This was my time to be with them, in the early months of their development. They needed me and I needed them. I knew when I returned to work, with all the travelling expected of me, there would be days I wouldn't get to see my children at all.

It was not a good place to be at the time and it has taken its toll. I have been left wondering why, on so many fronts, it is difficult to get justice, equality and fairness in this country. But I do take one positive thing from the whole debacle, something my GP said to me in the dark days: 'Try to turn this negativity around, try to turn it into something positive and enjoy your children while at home.' I did.

The organisation I worked for had lost all integrity and credibility in my eyes, and on that principle I would not return to work there. What may not be generally known is that because of the lack of legislation in Ireland, parents of children born through surrogacy have absolutely no statutory entitlement to maternity leave. Consequently, neither is there any entitlement to apply for additional statutory benefits such as unpaid leave following maternity leave, parental leave or term time. And we live in a country supposedly free from inequality and discrimination.

Despite the air of uncertainty and significant worry my work had inflicted upon us at this time, I tried to enjoy Christmas and make it pleasant for everyone. Regardless of all the efforts to bring upheaval and upset to our door, Santa did visit Donal and Ruby and Christmas was made even more special by having Diarmáid and Rián with us.

At some stage in the lead up to Christmas, Denise told us that the documentary was in the process of being edited and they would probably air it sometime in January. We were of course curious as to what the final programme would look like. Would it achieve what we had set out to do in the first place or would we regret agreeing to do it at all? We were also nervous about the local community and how they would react to the means by which we had achieved our family. Shortly into the new year, Denise phoned to say the date was set for Monday, 13 January. It would go out on RTÉ at 9.30 p.m. followed by a discussion on *Prime Time*. She and a colleague were going to travel down to us on the Wednesday beforehand to let us see the documentary in advance of it going out. That way at least we would be prepared for what was going to be in it. They were running a trailer the previous week on RTÉ, so by the first evening of the trailer going out, word had spread and the whole town seemed to know about the forthcoming documentary. By the time Wednesday came around there was a lot of nervous tension in our house as we sat down to see the final version, just Seán and I with Denise and her colleague. We had wine and beer to hand, in what was a weak attempt to quell the butterflies.

As the documentary unfolded, our faces displayed our emotional journey. We sat silently through it, experiencing a rollercoaster of emotions as we relived times and moments that brought hurt, sadness, joy and exhilaration. Afterwards we talked quietly about it. Overall we were pleased how sensitively and honestly our story had been depicted; certainly as much as could be achieved in the short sixty minutes.

51

HER BODY, OUR BABIES –
THE DOCUMENTARY

The closer the day loomed, the more nervous we became. We worried about the impact the documentary might have on us, on Donal and Ruby, on our community and on our families. It was the longest day ever waiting for 9.30 p.m. and even though we had seen it already we were still anxious and jittery about it going out on the national airwaves.

Emer, Mike and big Donal were coming over to watch it with us, and we felt it was an appropriate time to ask Donal and Emer to honour us by being godparents. They didn't hesitate, and I think I even saw a tear in Emer's eye. We also had Rián, Diarmáid and Mairéad asked, so there was plenty support for our lads if anything ever happened to us.

We knew watching it a second time wouldn't be any easier. There were bits we would have preferred not to be included, for example the unnecessary focus on our age which we felt only served to detract from the central topic of surrogacy. On the other hand, it showed very special moments: some that were full of fun and joy, but others that brought back the immense sorrow, pain and turmoil that surrogacy presents. For me the pain of our third baby dying to allow Donal and Ruby to live will never leave me. In the future, I know this will be difficult and painful to explain to Donal and Ruby. The making of the documentary is irrelevant to this; our intention was always to tell them the truth about where they have come from. Perhaps that will be the easy bit, but we have to tell them everything. We could never be dishonest with them. We just have to work out the how and the when and hope they understand the why. Our Aer Lingus flight coming in to land at Shannon was personally poignant for us, as we always felt that once home we could face anything together. Emer, Mike and Donal thought the documentary depicted surrogacy sensitively but realistically, and that we came across as being honest in our portrayal; we hoped so because we had laid ourselves bare in the name of honesty.

RTÉ had asked us to go on *Prime Time* following the documentary to discuss surrogacy and our experience. We declined, feeling the need to be at home with our family. We also wanted to take stock, see what kind of response the documentary invoked and consider our own response before any interviews. We knew we would generate a lot of discussion, and we certainly weren't naive enough to think we wouldn't be criticised. We would be exposing ourselves, showing our vulnerability, so we needed to wait. We needed to be prepared and strong enough for any media onslaught. We had no desire or willingness to go on every radio and TV show because doing that would only detract from and dilute our message, but we knew we would need to give some public interviews. We were aware the documentary would raise issues and pose more questions, which we would need to respond to, but also for us it was important to get across our reasons for making the documentary. Our intention was to choose carefully the few interviews we would do, try to reach as wide an audience as possible and tell the whole story.

People sometimes seem bemused, almost accusatory, when they ask why we made a documentary dealing with a topic that many find uncomfortable, even unpalatable and have difficulty understanding. Our original plan was to travel to India and return with a baby, if we were lucky enough, before people even knew we had left the country. We would say nothing; let people presume whatever they wanted: adoption, whatever. Instead we allowed ourselves to be exposed, with all our frailties and vulnerabilities, on national television to both accolade and denigration at the same time. We didn't do this for celebratory status, to make money or to depict ourselves as pioneers in this journey. Very simply, we wished to show people that alternative options exist. People should have access to this information and be allowed to make up their own minds as to whether they want to go the same road as us or not. I recall a comment I made early on in the documentary, 'It [surrogacy] is our last option but it is also the one giving us the most hope.' We wanted to give this hope to others.

Texts and calls started coming in once the programme had aired. One after the other, people expressed thanks and awe; some extoled our bravery and others simply wanted to let us know they supported us. *Prime Time* was as we expected, and we were glad we didn't agree to appear on it. A debate on surrogacy it was not. Unfortunately, the topic of surrogacy was lost in a debate about age and whether one had the right to have children in later years.

I didn't dare venture down town the day after. I wasn't ready to meet people yet. If truth be told, I was apprehensive. People needed time to take in what had been exposed on their TV screens; I needed time. I busied myself doing odd jobs around the house and looking after the lads. Sometime late morning I had a caller. Anne Rynne stood in my kitchen with her arms out to give me a hug, and what a welcome hug it was too! She simply said 'well done', and it was enough, exactly what I needed to hear at that time.

We expected some media attention but not the level we experienced in the days that followed. There was a lot of discussion on the radio and in the papers about it. Radio stations, newspapers and chat shows were all contacting us, seeking an interview. It was overwhelming. It wasn't all positive attention nor did we expect it to be. But no matter how strong or thick-skinned you are, when you become the subject of unkind personal comments you can find yourself in a very vulnerable place. In bed late one night, unable to sleep, I went onto the rollercoaster website. I was curious because earlier Mairéad had mentioned some negative discussion on it about us. She had actually been very kind because what I read was nothing less than a hate-filled, personal attack. Derogatory comments full of derision and venom were levied at us, in particular towards me. The comments were all anonymous, of course, made by cowardly people tapping out insults on a computer, too gutless to put their name to them. I made a mistake logging onto such websites. It was more important to focus on the reasons why we went public in the first instance. Our community rallying behind us, and all the letters, texts, cards and gifts we received reinforced our belief that we were right to go public. We had letters from people we didn't know, simply thanking us for giving them some hope when they thought they had none. These were the people we did it for and who in turn gave us the support we needed at the time. Those were the messages that were important. One simply said, 'unless you walk in my shoes'.

We knew the documentary cleared the way for discussion and debate which was good, that's what we wanted. A sixty-minute documentary was far too short to cover our journey through surrogacy, so we wanted to answer the questions that invariably were raised as a result. Most importantly, we wanted to get the government to do something about the issue instead of burying their head. They needed to be reminded time and again that children were being born every day through surrogacy, and they needed to be reminded that we could no longer tolerate such indifference to the issue; we needed legislation.

We had decided before the programme went out that, if asked, we would give one interview on national TV and one interview on our local radio station, Clare FM. Less was more; we didn't want to saturate the airwaves diluting the topic. Pragmatically, we considered what chat show reached the most viewers nationally, and based on that we decided to go on *The Late Late Show*. They wanted us on the following Friday night, and we had to agree to it being the first interview we would give. We received a call later, on behalf of RTÉ, asking us to do an interview for the *Sunday Independent*. We gave this over the phone for what was a series of articles being written on adoption. However, when the article appeared in the paper, our words had disappointingly been taken out of context and was not a clear reflection of our experience of surrogacy. Then some excerpts from that same article, along with photographs, appeared in other newspapers. It seemed they could share whatever they had on us without the common courtesy of telling us. This left a sour taste in our mouths, so we decided that where possible, we would only do live interviews. As such, what we said couldn't be taken out of context or misconstrued.

52

THE LATE LATE SHOW

*T*he *Late Late Show* beckoned and we all piled into a hired people carrier and headed for Dublin: Diarmáid, Rián and Annais, our au pair, accompanied me, Seán and the babies. After checking into the hotel, we had dinner with a glass of wine to settle the nerves. The plan was that Seán and I would go to the RTÉ studios first to get ready and meet with Ryan Tubridy, and the rest of our gang would follow on nearer to show time. We were picked up by taxi, led to our dressing room and given directions to make-up and the famous green room. After changing and having our make-up done we waited.

A knock on the door heralded the arrival of a smiling and pleasant Ryan Tubridy. He shook our hands in turn and put us at our ease quickly. He emphasised that we shouldn't be nervous or anxious, as the interview would be more an informal chat lasting about twenty minutes. He assured us that while the allocated twenty minutes sounded like a very long time, it would simply fly by. He assured us that if he asked anything difficult or if we got a mental block, we were not to worry. He would help us out of it; that was his job. He then went through the logistics. We would be first on after the show's final ad break, which would be about 11 p.m. Ruby and Donal would come on with us, and after the introductions they would be handed to Annais and Rián who would be in the front row of the audience.

It seemed straightforward, and we felt more relaxed after chatting to him, but still I couldn't help but wish it was over. The waiting was interminable that is until Rián, Annais, Donal and Ruby arrived shortly after, and we were kept busy until show time. Just as we headed towards the set, we were told of a change of plan. Donal and Ruby were not going on with us as previously arranged, instead they would be in the audience with Rián and Annais. We didn't object. We were too caught up about the interview to start pondering this change. As we were being led around the back of the set, we were told that we wouldn't be introduced onto the show like other guests; instead we would be in our seats when the ad break finished. On hindsight, these changes seemed to allow Ryan Tubridy to deliberately distance himself from what was a distasteful subject matter. Having Donal and Ruby in the audience as opposed to being with us on the set meant Ryan Tubridy did not have to introduce them or interact with them. This was in stark contrast to his other shows when he interacted at length with children.

One thing Ryan Tubridy did get right on the night was that once we were on the show, the twenty minutes flew by. The interview itself was not particularly easy, but then we didn't expect it to be. We wanted the difficult questions to be asked so that we could clarify issues for the public. What we didn't expect was the hostile manner of questioning. It was dogged and abrupt, and we knew we were not being given adequate time or opportunity to answer what was being asked of us. Again our age became an issue and particularly our right to have children at our age. We made the point that a man is never criticised or questioned about his age when it comes to fathering children, whereas a woman is constantly criticised if she happens to be over a certain age when becoming pregnant. Why is that? Ironically that same night, Red Hurley, who is over 65 years old and has a wife in her forties, appeared as a guest on the show. They had two children together, aged about 12 and 13. This meant that Red Hurley was about 52 – our age – when he had his children, but he wasn't taken to task by Ryan Tubridy and RTÉ. He certainly didn't demand the same scrutiny about his age as we seemed to. Disappointingly, the interview was not well balanced or fair towards us, and the line of questioning was definitely not objective.

Towards the end of the interview, the cameras swept briefly across Ruby and Donal – all too briefly and with no introductions. Once off camera, however, Ryan Tubridy did hold Ruby, albeit very briefly. We suspect it was for the audience's benefit because it certainly wasn't a genuine gesture towards us.

Seán was furious at how we were manipulated and how the line of questioning was an obvious attempt to undermine and discredit us publicly. I would say that only because Donal was out of sorts after the show and needed attention, he might have said something to Ryan Tubridy. While Seán walked the corridors of the RTÉ studios, I highlighted our dissatisfaction with one of the programme's producers. Contrary to Seán's belief, I felt we had handled ourselves pretty well under difficult circumstances. It was hard to assess how we presented ourselves. After we returned home, we watched the interview again and felt much better. We had answered every question thrown at us; we knew our subject and we were articulate in our responses. We had nothing to be ashamed of and nothing to berate ourselves about.

People at home came up to us on the street to tell us of how well we had spoken and responded to the line of difficult questioning. Many expressed anger at the way the interview had been conducted. On Monday, I listened to Ryan Tubridy's radio show and was surprised at the number of people who phoned in to say he had been quite unfair to us during the interview. They also questioned why he had not acknowledged Ruby and Donal during the interview. His response was a poor attempt at damage limitation. He said that people didn't see what happened off-air, and how he generally meets and chats with everyone in the green room after the show. As it happened, Ryan Tubridy did not meet with us or speak to us after the show, contrary to what was implied. In fact, we suspected he deliberately avoided us. In the aftermath, I wrote to RTÉ outlining our dissatisfaction at the way the interview was conducted.

Unsurprisingly, all we received was a standard letter of apology in response. We don't believe for one minute that anything is left to the last minute with meticulously executed chat shows like *The Late Late Show*. Everything about our appearance must have been planned and orchestrated well in advance; they just omitted to tell us of their plan.

Our second interview was on our own local radio station with Clare FM's John Cooke the following week. This interview was light years away from our unpleasant experience with *The Late Late Show*. His interview was impartial and objective. He posed some very difficult questions, but he was fair and importantly we were given time to answer. We were allowed to speak openly and honestly about the topic of surrogacy, and we were also able to clarify other issues that had been alluded to, for example, that we didn't get paid for any interview given to TV, radio or newspapers contrary to some public assumption. During this radio show the calls and texts that came in were diverse. Some were supportive while others were not, which is fine. Everyone is entitled to an opinion and we don't expect everyone to agree with us or agree with surrogacy. We respect that.

53

HELP AND HOPE

What was still amazing during this time was the amount of letters and cards we continued to receive from all over the thirty-two counties. The majority of the letters came from people we didn't know. They arrived daily. Some were simply addressed to 'the parents of Ruby and Donal', and others just had, 'Fiona Whyte and Seán Malone, Miltown Malbay' on the envelope. These messages from people all over the country reinforced our belief that we did the right thing in going public.

One of the letters struck a very strong chord with us. It read:

> Your beautiful babies are truly a miracle and it's lovely to see something good happen to good people. Sometimes we wonder what we have done to be so unlucky … I'm now 50 and it's time to give up on our dream, well really our future, as I believe your children are your futures. It makes us so sad deep inside our hearts, but we have to accept the situation and move on … Seeing your documentary we were amazed and thought if another couple from Ireland can make their dream come true maybe we have another chance … Hope this letter finds you for our sake, and if it has, thank you for taking the time to read it. We will be praying for an answer from you …Thanks so much for making the documentary, we would never have considered going to India but for you.

This couple are now a family since the birth of their son through surrogacy.

Another letter, this time from someone who is a parent to several children and is not considering surrogacy, said, 'You have advocated admirably on behalf of those involved in the world of surrogacy. So now sit lightly on the world and enjoy your son and daughter, you deserve it. Life goes on.' A couple, having gone through years of infertility, IVF and finally like us took the surrogacy path to have the baby they longed for, wrote, 'I've remembered your face and your parting answer on *The Late Late Show* when Ryan asked you if it was worth it and you said … Yes! I still cry with happiness for you both when I think of it as does my mam – and now I cry with happiness for us and we know it'll be worth it.'

These were simple words of thoughts and feelings from people who wanted to acknowledge the hope given in an Ireland which is so intolerant despite our times of change and progression – an Ireland where many are still struggling to experience the joy of being a father or a mother.

Some people went to extraordinary efforts to speak with us. One couple who phoned us had managed to get Seán's number by googling the pub. Another couple landed in Miltown one weekend on the off chance that they might come across us. They did and were successful in their quest. We gladly gave information to anyone who wanted it. We met many people and encouraged them on the journey. For as long as we continue to be asked, we will continue to give help and hope without hesitation or reservation.

What shocked us most were the numbers who had gone through the adoption process without any success. Even more shocking was that even after six, seven and eight years waiting, they were still hopeful of getting a baby. Some couples' declarations were running out, and they knew they faced a childless existence. Others were angry at a system that raised their hopes in a process that they now knew would never give them what they wanted most in the world. The reality of surrogacy is that people have a very real chance to have a child, to start a family. Is that so wrong?

On Christmas Day 2014 amidst everything we received an email from a couple whom we had encouraged and given information to about surrogacy. It read:

> A very happy Christmas to you both and to all your family. Thank you so much for your help and support. We have a tradition in our tiny estate in XXXX in the middle of nowhere where we bring together all eleven houses in our front garden and drink warm drinks and everyone brings goodies of some sort. Then we create a hundred and fifty lanterns out of brown paper bags, sand at the bottom to weigh them down and a tea light and we line the estate as a runway for Santa to let him know we are here and guide him in safely. Santa makes a brief appearance and gives a selection box to every boy and girl – Santa is my husband XXXX – I cry every year as Santa gives out the presents while keeping up external appearances of happiness. Today we had the joy of telling our neighbours our very happy news. It was lovely and I'm not sure it would have been possible without the two of you.

There will come a day when we will give Donal and Ruby all of these messages, all the cards, letters and emails sent to us so that we can reinforce the miracle of their being and help them to realise how precious they are, how wanted and absolutely loved they are.

54

WILL WE CHRISTEN?

One milestone in Ruby and Donal's life which caused much debate and consternation in our house was their christening. Seán being an atheist and I being a non-practising Roman Catholic, along with the revelations of child abuse in recent years within the Church, had caused us to seriously question whether we wanted the lads to be brought up as Catholic or not. Consequently, we were unsure if we wanted to christen them. I prefer to consider myself a spiritual person: we don't do wrong to anyone, we work hard and we live decent ordinary lives.

My older children and our au pair did not want us to have the traditional religious christening, as they felt we would only be hypocritical in doing so. Not entirely sure what direction to take, we tried to organise a humanist service or a naming ceremony as opposed to a religious event, but we didn't have any success in locating someone to do it for us. It seemed that we, in rural Ireland anyway, hadn't as yet embraced multi-denominational cultures. At the same time, we were acutely aware that our world will undoubtedly present difficulties for Donal and Ruby: because of their skin colour they will face ignorance, maybe hatred and most certainly discrimination in their lives.

By christening them there would be one less difference for them to deal with. We wanted to do the right thing, to make it easier for them not more difficult. All parents want that for their children. When they are old enough to decide for themselves, they can make their own decisions about the religious path or non-religious path they wish to take in life. Knowing our luck, one of them will want to enter a religious order or become a priest! But then if that happens then so be it.

We christened them the day Ireland was playing England in the rugby. After the service we would all return to the house where we would watch the game and have the usual knees-up with some tunes. Our family car was now much too small to accommodate everyone, so Seán had invested in a second-hand, nine-seater. On the day of the christening, we took it on its inaugural drive the short distance to the church. The service was nice and short, and Donal and Ruby behaved admirably throughout.

Mairéad had allowed me the privilege of borrowing the christening gown used by all her boys, and I also had the christening gown that I and my sons Diarmáid and Rián were christened in. Photographs and video recordings were courtesy of friends and then it was time to head home again in our red car. Half way to the house, as we led the cavalcade, disaster struck when our car started to backfire and splutter black smoke from its rear end. We barely chugged the last hundred meters home and were very lucky that we weren't walking or pushing it! But nothing could dampen our spirits that day for it was a day of celebrating their christening and of course Ireland beating England.

55

IRISH COURT PROCEEDINGS

On return to Ireland we had to apply to the Irish courts to ratify Seán's position as Donal and Ruby's legal guardian and custodian. Despite DNA results proving Seán to be the biological father and the Irish authorities issuing travel documents on that basis, there is still no entitlement under Irish law for Seán to be their legal guardian. The Irish Guidelines give a timeline of twenty working days by which one has to lodge the application to the Irish courts. We didn't do this within the required time frame, as quite simply we didn't have the cash. Prior to going to India we were quoted between €7,000–€8,000 plus VAT and barrister fees by a solicitor who was experienced in the area, so we figured the final bill was probably going to be in the region of €10,000 upwards.

Deferring our application was a precarious situation, as it meant Donal and Ruby didn't actually have any legal guardian in Ireland and the HSE were the only body legally entitled to consent or make decisions on behalf of our children. What if there was an emergency where one or other needed medical attention? What would happen if there was an accident? Would the HSE take responsibility? Who would we contact in the HSE if that was the case? What about out of hours, who in the HSE then assumed responsibility? No one had ever informed us of the HSE's responsibility towards Donal and Ruby while we awaited a court ruling. The precariousness of our situation was wholly endorsed by an indifferent government. The ironic bit about this is that while in India the Irish authorities had us jumping through hoops, reams of bureaucracy and red tape before being allowed home, yet on return it was as if we didn't exist. No government body or agency had contacted us since our return to ensure we complied with the Irish Guidelines or to check if we had even lodged court proceedings within the time frame.

When we were finally in a financial position to apply to the courts, we approached a local solicitor experienced in family law. We hoped by staying local we would be able to attend the local court, and maybe it would not be as expensive as initially quoted. We had all the documentation with us for our first meeting with Shiofra Hassett, and while she had no previous experience in dealing with surrogacy cases, Shiofra was confident she could represent us successfully. When she engaged her barrister, Marie Slattery, she arranged another meeting with us to discuss the case in more detail and outline how we would proceed. We liked them both and knew instinctively we had made the right choice. Shiofra was well prepared and had obviously researched the legal issues around surrogacy thoroughly. Marie exuded confidence; she was well experienced and capable. You would never have gleaned from them their lack of experience in dealing with surrogacy, as they confidently outlined the process for us and answered all questions. Our case would be heard in the Circuit Court in Ennis, and there would be two court appearances. The first was to serve the documents on the judge and get a hearing date; the second would be the day of the actual hearing itself. Marie advised that no application could be made on my behalf. The Attorney General would be represented in court by a solicitor to ensure the application was made on Seán's behalf only. The solicitor on behalf of the Attorney General would object to the application in its entirety if I pursued any legal entitlement. By all means I could attend the court, but there was no requirement for me to do so. I wasn't required; I didn't exist.

In advance of the first court appearance, Marie and Shiofra felt that while we had all of the required documents it might be prudent to seek an affidavit from Shobha's husband in relation to his marital status. It was an affidavit not on the list of required documents, but they felt it better to seek this now in advance rather than to be told in court we required it, delaying our case even more. On request, our Indian solicitor drew up the affidavit in English and Hindi and then arranged for Shobha's husband to sign it.

Once this was returned, we applied to the courts and received the date of our first appearance: 27 May 2014. It was a busy family-law day at the courthouse. People were milling about in the hallways, stairwells and anywhere there was an inch of space that could be utilised to discuss tactics. The building was bursting to the seams with solicitors and barristers. The media were skulking around corners scribbling notes about the ordinary Joe Soaps and their mundane lives. Some people were seeking custody, divorce or whatever while others prayed for their cases to be thrown out. Our hearing was estimated to be quite short, so we managed to get a slot in between some of the more lengthy hearings. It took all of fifteen minutes.

Standing before the judge, Marie had all the documentation prepared in book format and was ready for him. This appearance was exactly as predicted with the Attorney General represented by a solicitor who advised the court that the state would not object to Seán's application as long as I was not applying for any legal rights or entitlements. She stated that if I was making any application then the Attorney General had directed that an objection be lodged to the entire application.

Marie had also advised us that we might need to serve Shobha and her husband with a copy of the proceedings, despite Shobha having signed the affidavits waving all rights to Ruby and Donal. However, this was to be a decision for the judge at this hearing, and if it were the case, then there would be a time frame of six weeks allowed for Shobha and her husband to respond. There was a sense of urgency to our case which had never been lost on Shiofra and Marie, and it was now impressed upon the judge that Ruby and Donal could not continue to be left in legal limbo and without a legal guardian.

On hearing the details of our case, the judge ordered that proceedings be served on Shobha and her husband as predicted. He also agreed that Ruby and Donal should not be left in legal limbo and set a date for the hearing seven weeks later. We left the court with a date for 15 July 2014 for the full hearing, exactly seven weeks later. In the meantime, Shiofra would serve the proceedings on Shobha and her husband, giving six weeks to respond.

As expected, no response was received from Shobha and her husband. The family-law list on the day of our hearing was again extensive, but Shiofra and Marie were hopeful that we would get our case heard before some of the other more difficult cases. Instead of waiting around the corridors of the courthouse we were sent off for coffee with the promise that they would phone us when it was time for our hearing. A brisk walk up the town and two cups of coffee later, they were ready to hear our case.

We sat in the wings of an otherwise empty courtroom: the judge, Shiofra, Marie and the state's solicitor. We glanced around grateful to see that no reporters were present. Marie began by going through the proceedings, detailing each document for the benefit of the judge and the state solicitor. As times, some discussion ensued as she outlined and explained the various aspects of our application. Seán as the biological father was seeking a declaration of parentage as well as legal guardianship and custody of Ruby and Donal. If there was a court order granted to that effect, he was then seeking the right to apply for Irish passports for Donal and Ruby without having to acquire the consent of Shobha and her husband.

Coming to the end of the book of proceedings, Seán was asked to take the stand and was sworn in. Marie and Shiofra had prepared Seán in advance and now she repeated the same questions again. Inadvertently, he answered one question incorrectly. When asked what I worked at, he elevated me to the position of a 'director' no less. The judge followed on by asking the state solicitor if she had any objections to the application to which she confirmed she did not. The judge then ordered that as the DNA tests did prove Seán to be the biological father, he was entitled to have custody and be named as Donal and Ruby's legal guardian. The judge then ordered that Seán, on behalf of Donal and Ruby, could apply for Irish passports without having to seek Shobha and her husband's consent, until the age of eighteen at which time they could apply freely as adults. And that was it over, in so far as it could be under our current legal system.

Following the court order, Seán altered his will to appoint me as guardian intestate in the event of his death and to ensure that I would have the legal right to care for Donal and Ruby. Unfortunately that is the only legal provision that can be made for me as their mother. If this were not in place and if anything happened to him, then we would be back at square one with no legal guardianship for the lads. Of significant concern is that this provision does not cover the eventuality that Seán may become incapacitated; it only covers me in the event of his death.

56

CHANGING THE GOALPOSTS

As Donal and Ruby neared their first birthday celebrations, many of the couples we had met or given information to in the aftermath of the documentary were well into the surrogacy process in India. However, while the authorities continued to ignore the issue of surrogacy in Ireland, things had changed significantly in India in so far as the Irish authorities had made things a lot more difficult for Irish couples going to India for surrogacy.

There was no longer an Irish consulate in Mumbai, so people had to link directly with the Irish embassy in New Delhi every step of the way. DNA tests could no longer be carried out in Mumbai; instead they had to be carried out in New Delhi which meant people had to fly from Mumbai to New Delhi with a newborn baby for the DNA testing. This presented additional hardship and difficulties for the parents, as the airlines were reluctant to permit such young babies to fly. As a consequence, the airport authorities imposed their own requirements: the parents had to present a letter of discharge permitting a newborn baby to travel. Another issue arose in that as New Delhi was located in a different jurisdiction to Mumbai, another solicitor practising in New Delhi had to be appointed to notarise the documentation there. These changes were not notified in advance and only presented to those as they worked through the process. All this of course only served to add further stress and additional expense on people's pockets. It would appear to anyone looking in that the Irish authorities, rather than focusing their energy in introducing legislation in Ireland, were instead desperately trying to prevent Irish people from accessing surrogacy services in India.

While in India awaiting the emergency travel certificate for their newborn baby, another Irish couple told us how the goalposts had changed yet again for them. They had followed the Irish Guidelines to the letter, including every affidavit being translated into Hindi. But then they were informed that they not only had to do all that, but they also had to provide evidence that the surrogate mother could speak and understand Hindi. There was an inference that because the surrogate mother was from Mumbai she did not speak Hindi. The passport office were now saying the translations were incorrect, they wouldn't accept the terminology 'intended/biological' and they wouldn't accept that Hindi was the surrogate mother's language. A new problem had now been created by the Irish authorities, and it smacked of being awkward for awkwardness sake and reinforced the notion that there was a concerted effort to make it more and more difficult for Irish couples to access surrogacy services. Instead of safeguarding the rights of the child and their Irish parents, a smokescreen of ambiguity was instead being created.

The lads were doing everything they should have been doing as they reached their first birthday: walking, babbling, interacting and keeping us both busy and tired. Another milestone in their lives was reached, and we wouldn't have it any other way. Tomás settled into his role as a big brother, and while they drive him crazy when they throw toys all over the place, he is always gentle with them. Rián and Diarmáid help us out so much, relieving the pressure of looking after two live wires, always ready to jump in when asked. Now that Donal and Ruby are stronger and not as dependent, Marion is also very happy to spend hours playing peek-a-boo or ring-a-ring-a-rosy with them.

57

IRELAND'S LEGAL VACUUM

We still have no legislation in Ireland, and surrogacy still has no legal basis. Surrogacy remains neither legal nor illegal. In 2014, Minister Alan Shatter published a Heads of Bill, The Children and Family Relationship Bill, which went to the House of the Oireachtas. It recognised the diversity of families in all its forms, including surrogacy. It seemed to be moving in the right direction, but then suddenly Minister Shatter resigned, and the new Minister amended the bill to remove the section dealing with surrogacy. It is over ten years since the government's own Commission on Assisted Human Reproduction published its report in which it called on the government to introduce legislation on surrogacy. However, the state continues to fail to legislate and regulate surrogacy and assisted human reproduction (AHR) in Ireland. Despite the recommendations of the report, there isn't even guidance available to clinicians on AHR. Meanwhile, despite attempts to prevent Irish people from accessing surrogacy abroad particularly in India, surrogacy continues to happen and will continue to increase. We hear many speeches about what is in the best interest of the child. I often wonder when the government will realise that their denial and procrastination on dealing with the issue is not and cannot be in the best interest of the child.

2014 saw a Supreme Court ruling place the responsibility for introducing legislation in this area firmly on the shoulders of the legislators, our government. Successive governments have abdicated their responsibility in doing this, but the Minister for Health, Leo Varadkar, announced in mid-February 2015 that legislation on surrogacy and AHR would be drawn up and would be introduced. So where is it? While the Minister during interviews spoke of a consultative process, of draft legislation coming down the track and aspects of what might or might not be in the legislation, initial indications were vague and not specific enough to draw any conclusions as to how the legislation might look in reality.

In stark contradiction, then the Minister went on record to say that legislation would probably not be in place before the next general election in 2016, and the Taoiseach agreed. Why would the Minister go to the trouble of seeking consultation, drawing up legislation and then not implement it? The Irish government certainly cannot be accused of rushing this much-awaited legislation.

The following is a number of government proposals and our response to them:

- Minister Varadkar proposed to ban commercial surrogacy in all its forms. What will be allowed will only be altruistic surrogacy. No money will exchange hands except for reasonable expenses.

What are reasonable expenses? How will this area be monitored? When do reasonable expenses become a commercial fee? How does one compensate a woman reasonably for allowing her body to carry a couple's baby for nine months?

- The Minister proposed to introduce a contract based on consent. He has stated that the surrogate mother will have the opportunity to change her mind at any point during the pregnancy up to the point of 'Transfer of Parentage' in the courts.

How are the rights of the intending parents protected? What happens if one or both of the intending parents have a genetic connection to the baby and the surrogate mother changes her mind? Will this mean the intending parents, despite that genetic connection, have no legal rights while a surrogate mother who has no genetic connection retains all legal rights? Should the rights of all parties not be protected in a fair and balanced way? How will a surrogate mother be prevented from changing her mind in an effort to seek additional payments from the intending couple?

- The Minister has inferred that the intending couple will be assessed for 'suitability for parenthood'.

What will this look like? No information has been provided as to what this assessment will entail. The terminology in itself could be offensive to people who may already be parents. Is it acceptable that someone who gets pregnant unintentionally and is not in a position to care for a baby is not subject to assessment, whereas couples who may be parents already or who have been unable for whatever reasons to have a child are subject to rigorous assessment to determine their 'suitability'? Will this assessment process be similar to what is currently in place for adoptive parents? If so, will it continue to be a grossly intrusive and protracted process? While an assessment process may be required, it should not be a process based on elimination nor should it be a lengthy process taking several years which is currently the case for adoption.

- There may be an upper age limit included in the legislation. The government hasn't definitively stated what the age limit may be, but we know the upper age of 45 years has already been discussed.

It is not clear what the upper age limit will be nor how it will be determined. What are the grounds for having an upper age limit imposed on intending parents? A man can father children into his eighties while a woman can conceive naturally into her forties and even fifties. Why then would a 45-year age limit be imposed?

- The Minister stated that surrogacy will not be a service provided by the HSE; it will only be available to those who can pay for the service in a private capacity.

If a service is to be provided, should it not be available to everyone and not only for those who have money and can pay? Is this not commodification and commercialisation?

- The Minister also stated that surrogacy would only be available to couples who can provide a genetic link to the baby. Couples who require donor sperm and donor eggs will not be allowed to avail of surrogacy in this country. The Minister went further and stated that couples who went abroad for surrogacy services may on return to Ireland be guilty of committing an offence and face penalties.

Should surrogacy not be available to everyone irrespective of whether both donor eggs and sperm are required? At the moment surrogacy abroad is the only show in town, so should it not be factored into any new legislation to enable a seamless transition to a home-based surrogacy service? If people choose to go abroad for surrogacy services, how does the Minister envisage they be penalised on return and why? If surrogacy is legal in other jurisdictions, then why does the Minister state that Irish couples cannot legally avail of those services abroad? More importantly, couples will continue to go abroad to avail of surrogacy in other jurisdictions where surrogacy is legal if they cannot meet the criteria required in Ireland.

- The Minister made no mention as to how legislation will apply retrospectively to couples who have already had babies born through surrogacy either in Ireland or abroad. Will the parents and children be recognised in law? Will they be required to attend the courts again?

There should be provision in the legislation for retrospective recognition of the legal rights of parents and children born through surrogacy. Parents should not be subjected to having to go through another legal process with additional costs attached.

There remains much ambiguity and unanswered questions, and unless there is a consultative process undertaken and legislation addresses the diversity of the modern Irish family then we will be no better off than we are now. The government will continue to export the problem and people will continue to go abroad. We have a new minister now, Simon Harris, but still we remain in limbo.

EPILOGUE

In May 2015, Ireland was party to a particularly dirty referendum campaign on same-sex marriage. Both sides vigorously argued and debated their case. It was the 'No' campaign that seemed significantly more sinister in its use of dark tactics. We watched the RTÉ debate between Simon Coveney and Ronan Mullen, and it was the latter who caused us great offence when he asserted that 'the minute the surrogate mother gives birth, it is the last experience that baby will have of a mother's love'. Were we hearing right? How could anyone possibly say that? I relayed this comment afterwards to a mother whose baby had been born a few days previously through surrogacy. She replied by saying:

> It's amazing how years of hurt can be wiped away ... we had a tough night last night and I kept thinking how much better it is to have a rough night with an upset little one than the nights I've been awake worrying if we'd ever make it – I'm pinching myself still and I imagine I always will! It's so unfair to challenge the mother's love to a surrogate-born child that has gone on – I couldn't love XXXX more if I'd carried her myself and I will until my last breath!

Thankfully the Irish people in 2015 looked beyond their own existence and decided that everyone had a right to equality; that discrimination should not be given a seat at anyone's table and most importantly, that everyone is entitled to happiness in life. The referendum was carried. Maybe there is a chance in my lifetime that surrogacy will be legally recognised in Ireland, and that I will be legally recognised as my children's mother.

BBC WORLD NEWS: WEDNESDAY,
28 OCTOBER 2015

The Indian government has said it plans to ban surrogate services for foreigners. In response to a Supreme Court request to the Indian government to set out its plans for regulating surrogacy, the government has responded in an affidavit to the Supreme Court that surrogacy will only be made available to married, infertile, Indian couples. They plan to introduce this in law, but as it will take some time, all clinics have been requested to hold all surrogacy cases temporarily. December 14, 2015 was the day the shutters descended on foreign surrogacy in India, and unless already in the process at that date, it was the end of the road for many hopefuls.

EMAIL TO OUR SOLICITOR, SHIOFRA HASSETT:
18 MARCH 2016

Hi Shiofra, hope you don't mind me emailing you.

I have looked at the new Children and Family Relationship Bill 2015 and specifically under PART 4, Section 45 6C and I feel I can apply to the courts for guardianship of Donal and Ruby, as I meet the criteria outlined within Section 45 6C (1) and (2).

I don't know whether this is a loophole, intentional or otherwise, but would you have a look at it for me and advise if we can pursue this avenue to ratify my position as the legal guardian of my children?

Many thanks in hopeful anticipation,

Fiona and Seán

CHILDREN AND FAMILY RELATIONSHIP BILL 2015

PART 4

Section 45 6 C (1) *The court may, on an application to it by a person who, not being a parent of the child, is eligible under subsection (2) to make such application, make an order appointing the person as guardian of a child.*

(2) A person is eligible to make an application referred to in subsection (1) where he or she is over the age of 18 years and –

(a) on the date of application, he or she –

    (i) is married to or is in a civil partnership with, or has been for over 3 years a cohabitant of, a parent of the child, and

    (ii) has shared with that parent responsibility for the child's day-to-day care for a period of more than 2 years.

Shiofra's advice was that we could and should bring an application. The only uncertainty was whether we would need to join Shobha and the Attorney General to the proceedings as we had done before. The preference was to just have myself as the applicant and Seán as the respondent, to expedite matters and keep things as simple as possible. But if we didn't serve Shobha and put her on notice, the court might decline to deal with our case. As the respondent, Seán would also have to be served and put on notice.

In December 2016, Shiofra initiated the process to have me appointed a legal guardian of our children by lodging the draft proceedings with the District Court Office. I was the applicant in the proposed proceedings while Seán and Shobha were the proposed respondents. The first step was to seek the court's permission to issue and serve the relevant proceedings outside of the jurisdiction, i.e. India. Shiofra made this application on 2 December to Ennis District Court. If our case could be heard in the District Court as opposed to the Circuit Court, it would also be less costly for us as we would not need to appoint a barrister. The judge, however, was reluctant to deal with proceedings in the District Court, given that related proceedings had been dealt with in the Circuit Court. Shiofra's view was that those proceedings were finalised, and that these were new proceedings under new legislation, but the judge wanted to consider the matter until 15 December.

Our hearing was finally set for 16 February 2017 in the District Court. We arrived at 10.30 a.m., searching for Shiofra through that day's mass of dour-faced family-law applicants and respondents. Taking us aside, she quickly went through the process: our case would be put on the short list, meaning it would be a short case and should be dealt with quickly. I may or may not be sworn in and questioned; if sworn in, then Shiofra would take me through the questions. Shiofra hesitated, looking at us with concern etched on her face, and said there was no guarantee we would come away with a result today. The judge could decide during the hearing that it was a case for the Circuit Court, given that this application was in relation to surrogacy and, as far as we were aware, it would be a first of its kind, and would, most importantly, set precedence. Or the judge could reserve his judgement for a future date – or maybe we would be refused altogether.

The latter we didn't dwell on. Shiofra confirmed she had served Shobha and, as expected, no response had been received. She hadn't served the Attorney General as we were not applying for anything outside of this new legislation. She then said that she hadn't served Shobha's husband, either. This caused me a pang of anxiety as I immediately felt that this was a mistake, but Shiofra, in her confident manner, explained that as the previous proceedings had established Seán to be the biological father, thus granting parentage to him, there was no reason to serve Shobha's husband. Somewhat appeased but not sufficiently to feel confident, we sat down to wait for our case, number 19, to be called.

'Case number 19, FW and SM please.' Shiofra emerged from the innards of the long hall to nod at us and we moved to the court room. Seán sat up towards the front while I sat behind Shiofra. No one else was there except for the lone Garda on duty, a couple of court staff and the inevitable reporter or two looking bored and lonesome in the corner. Shiofra started by stating the legislation under which the application was being made, and then outlined the application. The judge confirmed I was the applicant and told me to take the stand. I was sworn in, gave my name and address, and answered Shiofra's questions one by one.

How long was I in a relationship with Seán? When were Donal and Ruby born? Where were they born? Was I present at the birth? Did I return to Ireland with Seán, Donal and Ruby? Have I cared for my children since arriving back to Ireland? Do we reside together at our home? All questions answered, the judge excused me and I returned to my seat to wait.

The judge asked Seán if he had any objection to my application ... none whatsoever.

He started reading the order and I realised it was happening ... and so it was granted. In a matter of ten minutes I was, at long last, by court order, the legal guardian of our children. I couldn't keep the beaming smile off my face and everyone followed suit, the Garda, Shiofra and the staff, while Seán was both smiling and teary-eyed with emotion. Shiofra said afterwards that we were probably the only people who left court smiling that day. Just before we exited, the judge turned and wished Seán, myself, Donal and Ruby all the best for our future. This was the long-sought acknowledgment that we were a family, and one finally recognised in Irish law.

We no longer needed to worry about what would happen if Seán became incapacitated – the lads would have had no legal guardian – and what if one or other of the children had an accident and Seán wasn't around – at least now I can consent for them. This outcome was the best we had hoped for, the best we could hope for in the absence of any legislation.

We have now come to the end of the road; we have gone as far as we can go for our beloved and beautiful children. The rest is up to the Irish State and those who propose to act on our behalf, and on behalf of all the citizens of Ireland.

Donal and Ruby are those Irish citizens – without a shadow of a doubt.